Praise for *Savasana*

Savasana: Between Breath and Death offers grace, moments of being—and of being other. It grants permission to let go. I found myself soulfully wrapped in this guide by Leslie Howard and Richard Rosen, drawn to its invitation to explore a quieter, more contemplative side of death work, which I thought I knew intimately—and the yogic wisdom I now yearn to explore more deeply. I recommend it.

    Erin Oliver, Supervisor Operations, Hospice Volunteer Services, Kaiser Permanente

Leslie Howard's work on savasana offers a vital contribution to the field of yoga studies and integrative health. She demonstrates with clarity and precision how the deliberate practice of stillness provides access to profound interoceptive and contemplative states. In a society marked by overstimulation and constant outward engagement, this book highlights the therapeutic significance of deep rest—not as passive withdrawal, but as an active, transformative process of self-awareness and restoration. It is an essential resource for clinicians, scholars, and practitioners alike.

    Amy Wheeler, PhD, chair, Yoga Therapy and Ayurveda Dept., Notre Dame of Maryland University, School of Integrative Health

This wonderful book is a timely and welcome gift. At first glance, it is an inspiration to stay in your yoga class till the end and rest, to enjoy savasana, the corpse pose. It also invites us to consider all the aspects of savasana: to disentangle from the thinking that we are our bodies, the invitation to see ourselves as an eternal Self like a never-fading light, to become more comfortable with the truth of our last breath, and much more. Yoga teachers will learn much about teaching and propping this pose as well.

    Annie Carpenter, founder of SmartFlow Yoga

(continued on next page)

Finally, the quintessential book on the most important pose of the 21st century, *Savasana: Between Breath and Death*, written by two of the leading yoga researchers and practitioners, Richard Rosen and Leslie Howard. In a world that is loud, restless, and violent, it is difficult to be still, listening, and content; and yet what could be more important and fulfilling? What is the history of this posture, its original purpose, and how does that translate to the present day? All of that is served to you in this book with humor and practicality. Basically, a survival manual that leads to joy and freedom.

    Rodney Yee, yoga teacher and author

This book is fantastic. I learned a lot from it, and it inspired a wonderful savasana experience. *Savasana: Between Breath and Death* is a work of wisdom, dedication, and love. Take its lessons to heart; they will enhance your savasana, and your life.

    Roger Cole, sleep scientist and yoga teacher

This is a timely book and practical book, eminently useful to both students and teachers. Leslie and Richard's comprehensive yet direct work, which teases out the many dimensions of this practice, reminds and enlightens us as to what yoga is, and—as the title suggests—how it can be made a constant companion.

    Doug Keller, yoga teacher and author

I still remember my first yoga practice and the first savasana that kept me coming back for more. Now, with this accessible, thoughtful work by Leslie Howard and Richard Rosen, we can all go way beyond that first taste of savasana and dive into the richness it offers.

    Baxter Bell, MD, coauthor of the book *Yoga for Healthy Aging*

Howard and Rosen invite readers to explore how practicing savasana opens a pathway to insight within the body and mind, granting access to a deeper awareness of mortality and meaning that we can carry off the mat and into life.

    Francesca Lynn Arnoldy, author of *Kindred Grief Care*
    and *Cultivating the Doula Heart*

SAVASANA

SAVASANA

Between Breath and Death

LESLIE HOWARD & RICHARD ROSEN

© 2026 Leslie Howard and Richard Rosen

All rights reserved. No part of this publication may be reproduced, distributed, or transmitted in any form or by any means, including photocopying, recording, or other electronic or mechanical methods, without the prior written permission of the author, except in the case of brief quotations embodied in critical reviews and certain other noncommercial uses permitted by copyright law.

Leslie Howard
lesliehowardyoga@gmail.com
www.lesliehowardyoga.com

This book is not intended as a substitute for the medical advice of physicians. Readers should regularly consult their physician in matters relating to their health and particularly with respect to any symptoms that may require diagnosis or medical attention.

ISBN: 979-8-218-89493-1 (paperback)
ISBN: 979-8-218-89494-8 (e-book)

First Edition
30 29 28 27 26 | 10 9 8 7 6 5 4 3 2 1

Book design and composition by BookMatters, Berkeley
Photographs by Hannah Moss
Cover design by James Aarons
Cover art by Katarzyna Kopańska

CONTENTS

Foreword — ix
TIAS LITTLE

Preface — xiii

How to Read This Book — xv

PART I **The Pose**

1. What Is Yoga? — 3
2. Savasana: The Basics — 9
3. Savasana: Getting in, Getting out, Modifications and Variations — 12
4. How to Be in Savasana — 48
5. The Still Point on the Path: Effort and Surrender — 51
6. How to Exit Savasana: Because That's Just How I Roll — 54

PART II **Supportive Practices for the Restless and the Dying**

7. The Breath: Pathway to Stillness — 61
8. Mantra: The Sound That Carries Us Home — 66
9. Mudras: Yoga in Your Hands — 69

PART III	**Death**	
10	The Pose That Reveals the Path	81
11	The Liminal Space: Coming Home	87
12	Practice Dying and Do It in Savasana	91
13	Let the Reaper out of the Closet	94
14	The Death Positivity Movement	94

Epilogue   107

Appendix: Teaching Savasana (For Teachers and the Just Plain Curious)   111

   Key Reminders for Every Practice   112

   Adjusting Your Students   112

   Words Matter   115

   Cueing Styles   116

   Sample Savasana Scripts   117

   Bringing Students out of Savasana   120

Book Club Questions   123

Acknowledgments   125

Index   127

About the Authors   131

To all of our teachers, and our teachers' teachers—

but especially to Ramanand Patel,

who has been our yoga beacon in this life and, hopefully, the next.

FOREWORD

It is fair to say that savasana, the "pose of the corpse," is the most important of all yoga postures. The classic Buddhist text, the *Parinirvana Sutra*, declares "of all meditations that on death is supreme." The big irony is that while seemingly inert and static, savasana is actually a dynamic and vivifying pose meant to restore the body's essential life force.

While most classes save it for last, like a crème brûlée off the dessert menu, I prefer to start my classes in savasana. Many do not realize that savasana is a practice in and of itself. This is in keeping with the foundational teachings of the Buddha, who encouraged four positions for meditation:

- Sitting
- Standing
- Walking
- Lying down

Lying down may be the optimal orientation—when the body is horizontal, supported by the ground and released from gravity, any stored resistance in the musculature, organs, joints, and bones goes slack. Physiologically, savasana works like a kind of sleep, regenerating the nerves, glands, and cells of the body. Psychologically, savasana is a blueprint for letting go.

This is in keeping with one of the fundamental tenets of yoga: In order to experience a boundless, undifferentiated, unified state of being, we must first relinquish the "clench" in our bodies and minds. Ultimately, savasana is an invitation to let go of who you think you are and who you think you ought to be.

In the stillness of savasana, there is an entire universe to explore. It is a position of "active rest," a dynamic stillness that, for the initiated, offers a remarkable glimpse into the fundamental nature of consciousness. While not outwardly moving, we encounter, just under our skin, an entire ecosphere of breath, sensation, pulses, secretions, waves, and electrical currents. Like seated meditation, it is a position that allows for a rich exploration of the inherent, life-sustaining gift of prana, the breath of life.

Savasana is a threshold pose. It takes us into a gap, a bardo, a liminal space between life and death. The direct experience of savasana mirrors the end of life. Perhaps you have had the opportunity to sit, bedside, next to a loved one who has entered the tunnel of death. The moment is powerful, astonishing, unforgettable. In the half-light between living and dying, the entire room becomes still. It is a rarefied atmosphere, like the air following a big storm that suddenly becomes completely motionless, devoid of any wind.

When confronting the immensity of death, we realize that we are just tiny specks in an infinitely vast space, one without boundary, edge, or seam. In that narrow opening, a small rift in the flimsy veil separating life from death, we experience a strange wonder. Any direct glimpse of death leaves us with a renewed appreciation for this precious, tenuous, ephemeral human life.

Savasana: Between Breath and Death is an invaluable guide into the very essence of the yoga teachings. This book is a plunge into the mysterious presence of the vital force that sustains us all. It is a template for navigating a realm that is inherently beyond measure and outside our grasp. In death's doorway, in the embodiment of savasana, the most we can do is to rest in the unknown and to open ourselves to an impossible grace.

When we are deeply relaxed in savasana, we enter a realm beyond calculation. In the process of dying, reason loses traction. And when reason loses traction, the possibility of faith arises.

The practice of savasana is, by necessity, a process of unselfing.

Like a snake shedding its skin we must slither out from under our beliefs, our identity, and any attempt we might muster to grasp what is happening. In the depths of savasana, the most we can do is relinquish ourselves to the immeasurable and maybe, just maybe, encounter on the other side of the veil of "me," a great and enduring peace.

Tias Little
SANTA FE, NEW MEXICO

PREFACE

> **Lying on the Earth on your back like a corpse is savasana. Savasana removes fatigue and brings rest to consciousness.**
>
> —*HATHA YOGA PRADIPIKA* 1.32
> (15TH CENTURY CE), SVATMARAMA

> **Death is something that can be just as easily done while lying down.**
>
> —WOODY ALLEN

Savasana is one of the most underappreciated poses in yoga. Often practiced at the end of class, it's mistakenly viewed as a simple relaxation exercise. Many think that "real" yoga demands focus, energy, and balance, while lying still seems little more challenging than taking a nap. Why bother?

Yet in traditional yoga philosophy, savasana holds deep significance. The name itself, *sava* meaning "corpse" and *asana* meaning "seat," suggests a profound purpose. We suspect that the holy men of yoga, and most traditional yogis were men, chose the name precisely because of the psychological and physical weight it carries. Renowned yogi B.K.S. Iyengar called it the most difficult pose, requiring complete surrender of both body and mind.

This book explores savasana in depth: as a pose, as a path, and as a preparation for death. Practically, it enhances health and well-being. Symbolically, it's a rehearsal for our final "exit." In Western culture, death is often ignored or feared. In yogic understanding, it's an opportunity for liberation, letting go of ego and embracing life more fully.

We hope to convince you that savasana is one of the most significant poses and that it does not always get the attention it deserves. We will cover the full depth and breadth of savasana, from its nuts and bolts, to its transformative mental and physical effects, to its role in confronting mortality.

Savasana is both a down-to-earth everyday practice and a symbolic "rehearsal" for that final curtain call. In much of Western culture, death is the price we pay for being alive. In yogic philosophy, savasana is the practice of dying. By turning toward death, we begin to see that what we most fear can also reveal life's greatest beauty. The simple act of lying still on the floor has the potential to utterly transform our lives.

In gratitude,
Leslie and Richard

HOW TO READ THIS BOOK

Readers will come to this book from different doorways. You may be a longtime yoga student curious about more nuanced savasana experiences. You may be a teacher wanting to offer your students a deeper practice in the final pose. Or you may be someone outside the yoga world altogether, drawn here by questions about mortality, the Death Positivity movement, or end-of-life care.

Wherever you begin, here are some suggestions:

- FOR YOGA TEACHERS: Read the whole book if you can for practical ways to enrich your teaching. Don't miss the Appendix, which offers strategies for guiding savasana, language tips, and sample scripts.
- FOR YOGA STUDENTS: Begin with chapters 1–6 to gain a clear understanding of what savasana asks of you—and why "doing nothing" can be the most radical practice of all.
- FOR THOSE INTERESTED IN DEATH AND DYING: Head directly to part II—Supportive Practices for the Restless and the Dying on death and dying, where we connect savasana to end-of-life awareness, death positivity, and liberation teachings.

This book is not meant to be rushed. You might move through it linearly, or circle back to passages again and again. However you read it, may it meet you where you are—in practice, in teaching, and in life.

PART I
The Pose

1 | What Is Yoga?

If we searched all our yoga books for a definition, we'd find more variations than we could count. Yoga is often called a "philosophy." But for Westerners, that term can be misleading. In the West, philosophy is mostly intellectual—thinking, debating, writing papers. Yoga, however, is an "embodied philosophy," where theory becomes action: breath, movement, stillness, and sensation. You don't just think it, you live it. There are no existentialist headstands or stoic downward dogs.

That's not to say there is no thinking in yoga. Every traditional school of yoga comes with a robust theoretical backbone, which could be called a philosophy, about the nature of the world, the self, and what lies beyond.

Yoga has no single, definitive view of the world or the self. Instead, it offers a wide variety of schools, each appealing to different people and contexts. Today's most popular styles are hybrids that blend traditional Hatha yoga, whose roots date back to the 15th century, with modern adaptations. In the 21st century, yoga has expanded into countless forms, from fast-paced flows to gentle restorative classes, serving every age and ability.

The roots of Hatha yoga go back to the mid-1400s when postures, including a version of savasana, enter the picture in recognizable form. Many other poses were adapted from other body-movement systems, such as calisthenics, military conditioning, and gymnastics.

Fast forward to the here and now. Yoga has taken off in ways the old yogis never could have imagined. There are fast flow classes and gentle ones; classes for toddlers, teens, and seniors; yoga for pregnancy, for recovery, for pelvic floors, for people with disabilities—you name it. It's our good fortune to be living in a time when yoga truly is for everyone.

A Brief History of Savasana

The earliest record of savasana appears in the 13th-century Dattatreya's *Discourse on Yoga*, though the practice likely predates the text. Originally, savasana was a *samketa*, an esoteric technique, within Laya yoga, a practice of dissolution. By the mid-15th century, this technique was transformed into an asana.

Traditional texts were brief, as yoga was taught in person by gurus and kept secret from the uninitiated. Later works, like the 18th-century *Hatha Tatva Kaumudi*, offered slight variations, describing specific positioning, meditation on Shiva, and benefits for body and mind.

Only in the 20th century did detailed written instructions emerge, as yoga moved into the public sphere. Teachers like Shri Yogendra (1897–1989) devoted entire sections of their books to savasana, marking a shift toward written guidance as the main teaching method.

This samketa appears again in the mid-15th–century compilation *Hatha Yoga Pradipika*, an organized patchwork of unattributed excerpts borrowed from other, usually older, texts. Today, such a method might be labeled plagiarism, but in India at the time it was a common practice; spiritual knowledge was considered the collective inheritance of the community, to be shared freely. Interestingly, the *Hatha Yoga Pradipika* re-imagines the samketa as an asana—specifically, savasana:

> Lying supine on the ground like a corpse—that is savasana.
> Savasana wards off fatigue and brings mental repose. (HP 1.32, translation by Kaivalyadhama)

The brevity of this description should not be mistaken for a lack of importance. Almost all traditional yoga texts present asanas in the fewest words possible. Yoga was, after all, a guarded discipline, taught only to initiated students, typically in person by a (male) guru. Written accounts were meant as brief reminders, not as step-by-step instructions. We will likely never know exactly how these postures were practiced in their original form.

Most of the texts following the *Hatha Yoga Pradipika* (that we had access to) up to the beginning of the 20th century simply copied the instruction from the HP without attribution or elaboration. But there is a written description of savasana in an 18th-century text, the *Hatha Tatva Kaumudi* (*Moonlight on the Principles of Hatha*, hereafter HTK) by the modestly named Sundara Deva, "handsome god," that gives some variation. HTK states:

> Lie on the ground in the supine position, legs apart, place the folded hands on the chest, gaze fixed at the tip of the nose, meditate on Shiva. This is savasana. Practice of savasana cures the knots (obstructions) caused by vitiated *Vata* in the chest—that is, disturbances in the body's air and movement principle, often associated with restlessness or nervous tension—and removes the fatigue of the body-mind arising due to the practice of all the asanas and exhaustion. This brings well-being to the yogi. All the asanas like *siddhasana*, *padmasana*, lead to success in yoga, bring rest to the tired body…rest to the "consciousness" (*citta*) happens on lying, and *citta* becomes poised. (7.11–13)

Only as we enter the 20th century do asana instructions become more detailed, a shift driven by the practice moving into the public arena and away from the individualized, guru-to-disciple model. As yoga began to reach wider audiences, especially in the West, the direct encounter between teacher and single student became less common. A new era in yoga instruction was born: the written word became the teacher.

As a result, descriptions of asanas expanded dramatically in both length and detail. One of the earliest examples is *Yoga Asanas Simplified*, first published in 1927 by the "householder yogi" Shri Yogendra. Remarkably, it devotes a full five pages to savasana. A noteworthy aside: Sita Devi, Yogendra's spouse, published the first

> **A Note on the Text**
>
> When we convert Sanskrit into English, we're either translating (changing meaning) or transliterating (changing script). Transliteration from the Devanagari alphabet, which has around 46–48 characters, to our 26-letter Roman alphabet presents challenges, especially with consonants like sibilants. Devanagari has three "s" sounds, while English has only one. So scholars use diacritical marks to distinguish them. For example, the palatal "s" (made by pressing the tongue to the roof of the mouth) is written as ś. This comes into play with the word *savasana*, which is often mispronounced as SAH-VAH-SAH-NAH or spelled shavasana to guide English speakers toward the more accurate pronunciation, SHAH-VAH-SAH-NAH. Technically, the correct transliteration is śavāsana, but using diacritics throughout would have made the book less accessible. For clarity and consistency, we chose the more familiar spelling: savasana.

yoga instruction book for women in 1934, and it is still in print today.

Ever-Evolving Savasana

Hatha yoga as a whole underwent significant changes as it entered the 20th century and spread to the West. From a survey of 10 yoga instruction manuals published between 1904 and 1968, we can identify no fewer than four innovations in the presentation of savasana, alongside a dramatic increase in the amount of detail given for its performance.

Variations

The pose begins to appear in multiple forms. Some teachers suggest it be performed prone or lying on one side. For example, Shri Yogendra describes a posture he calls *Dridhasana* ("firm, strong"), in which the practitioner lies on the right side, using the right arm as a "pillow" (Yogi Gupta, *Yoga and Long Life: The Basic Principles of Hatha Yoga*, p. 124). This, he claims, improves both digestion and

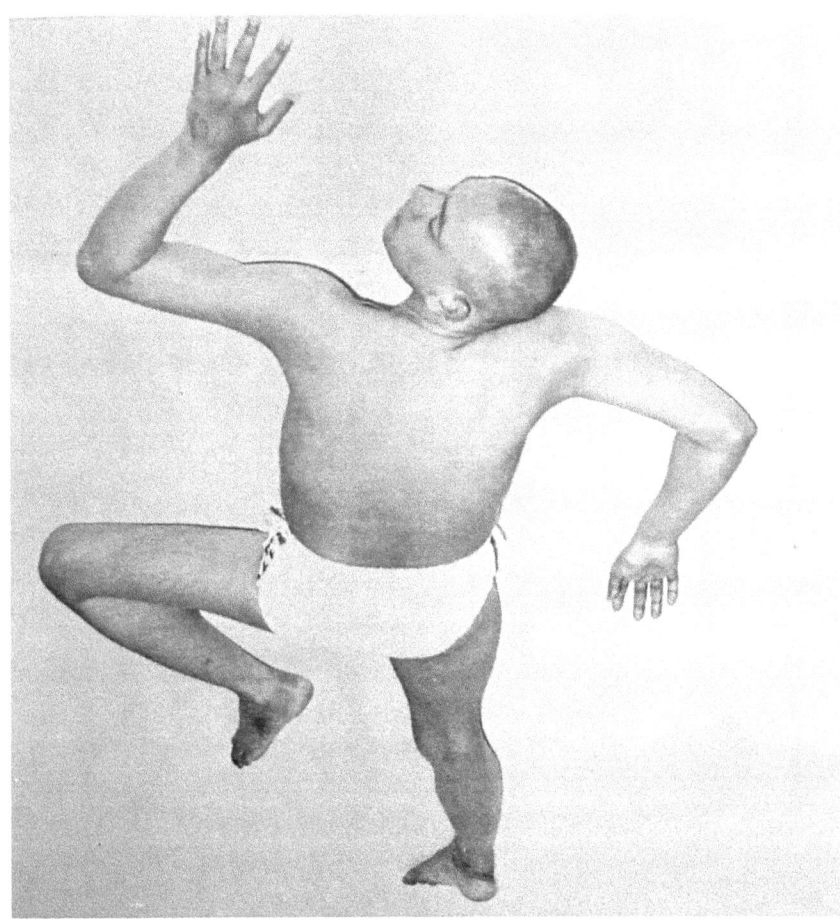

Yogi Gupta (1913–2011) in a prone form of savasana, placing the body in what appears to be an unusual position, yet one he personally prefers for "relaxing."

breathing. Another Yogendra variation has the practitioner lying on the belly (prone), in a posture he named *Makarasana*, usually translated as "Crocodile," though more properly "Sea Monster." In modern yoga, *Makarasana* is often taught as a variation of *Salabhasana* ("Locust," see B.K.S. Iyengar, *Light on Yoga* [LoY], p. 100). But traditionally it was a resting pose: the forehead supported on crossed forearms, legs spread wide, and feet turned onto their inner edges (everted, see Gheranda Samhita 2.40).

Yogi Gupta (1913–2011) also presents a prone form of savasana, placing the body in what appears to be an unusual position, yet one he personally prefers for "relaxing" (Yogi Gupta, p. 144).

For us, it's hard to see how this pose is relaxing, but it may be just the position you need. Alternatively, Gupta describes the usual supine position. He also notes that "one may practice relaxation sitting in a chair or standing in the street" (Yogi Gupta, 144).

Visualization

Visualization introduces simple internal images to quiet the mind. The "English yogi" Ernest Wood recommends "thinking upon something pleasant." Indra Devi, a pioneer of yoga as exercise, offers the more poetic "a soft white cloud drifting in the sky" (*Yoga for You*, p. 75).

Progressive Relaxation

Progressive relaxation involves imaginatively directing the breath into and out of a set sequence of body parts. Approaches may vary, but the progression typically begins with the big toes and ends at the crown of the head. The yogi Yogacharya Sundaram calls this technique "auto-suggestion" and attributes it to the ancient Indian text known as the Vedas (around 1500 BCE), although he doesn't cite a specific source.

Timing

The timing of savasana has changed in two ways. Traditionally, it seems that savasana was performed only as a part of an asana practice. Now, it can be a stand-alone practice. There is no clear history on when savasana should take place, traditionally, as part of the asana cycle or at the end of the asana cycle. Now, savasana is the caboose at the end of the asana train.

How can this brief history of savasana inform our practice?

First, it is an asana. It needs to be practiced consistently over time with patience to gain from its full range of health-giving benefits.

Second, it is not static. Modern yoga has expanded the ways in which the pose can be practiced, especially with the addition of yoga props.

Third, it is timeless. Savasana has moved into the mainstream culture, with application for a spectrum of physical and psychological needs for yogis and non-yogis.

2 | Savasana: The Basics

Savasana's role is to settle down, digest, and assimilate the practice, to experience resonance. It is a time of absorption, absorbing and being absorbed.

—FRANÇOIS RAOULT

What's So Hard about Lying Down?

How many nuts and bolts are necessary for a pose that essentially consists of lying on the back for a few minutes with the eyes closed? We often make the mistake of believing that, in order for a pose to be considered a "real" asana, it must induce us to do something. But savasana is like a vinyl record, it's the "flip side" of all the other asanas. Instead of doing something, the point is to do nothing.

Movement Beyond the Physical

Movement is generally physical; a swinging arm or leg. Yogis contend that thinking is also movement. How so?

We tend to talk about "my body" and "my mind" as if they are two separate realities, a dualism. We apply that to the entire world, I am "in here" and everything else is "out there."

The yogis see the world as a single reality: *Tat tvam asi*, or "I am That." If our body is moving, so is our mind. In savasana, we're encouraged to keep our bodies as still as possible, like a corpse, in order to still our minds. If our minds are still active—that is, still thinking—then we are, in effect, still moving. This mental movement is a much greater obstacle to corpse pose than physical stillness. The reason savasana is radically different from even the most relaxing nap is that during the latter our minds remain active; they wander, dream, move.

B.K.S. Iyengar said that "it is much harder to keep the mind than the body still. Therefore, this apparently easy posture [savasana] is one of the most difficult to master" (*Light on Yoga*, p. 422).

The Paradox of Effortless Effort

If savasana requires the cessation of all movement and we are asked to still our minds, isn't the deliberate effort to *stop* everything still a movement? Isn't the act of stilling the mind also a mental activity? Perhaps it's becoming a little clearer the challenge that savasana the asana presents.

A Pose in Three Acts

All poses, savasana included, have three stages: A beginning, a middle, and an end. Students often focus on just the middle stage, the pose itself. But every pose is more like a movie, not just a single frame. Entering and exiting poses properly is crucial. The entry has a significant influence on our experience in the pose; the exit affects our experience after the pose. Our "nuts and bolts" will cover all three stages, including what to do and what not to do.

The revitalization of yoga at the beginning of the 20th century brought savasana innovations. Here, we offer many tried and true variations of corpse pose, suitable for either countering or creating a variety of conditions.

Classic supine savasana, and its variations, include props. You may not be accustomed to props beyond a yoga mat and a blanket. Traditionally, savasana was practiced without props. Perhaps props were not readily available or they weren't needed. (It's highly unlikely ancient yogis were grappling with "tech neck"!) If there was discomfort in classic supine savasana, maybe it was seen as part of the practice, an element to be observed, tolerated, or transcended.

Supportive props can help us, in our modern-age bodies, access deeper states of rest and awareness. We strongly believe that belts, sandbags, blankets, bolsters, and more are a useful practice supplement. If you don't have props at hand, feel free to improvise, a bathrobe belt or old necktie can become a yoga belt, rolled up blankets or towels can become a bolster. Have the props nearby and try different setups to see which one gives you the clearest path into stillness.

Beyond the Asana Train: Stand-Alone Savasana

Savasana is no longer just the caboose of the "asana train." It's a three-stage pose in its own right and the use of props can prepare the body for a longer stay in the pose. Simultaneously, corpse can be taken "off the mat," that is, done independently of an asana practice for a variety of reasons, such as stress management, insomnia relief, or simply for relaxation.

3 | Savasana
Getting in, Getting out, Modifications and Variations

Classic Supine Savasana

Overview

This pose can be done by itself anytime to relax or as a way to start or end a yoga session. Once you are set up, we recommend at least 10–15 minutes. Please note this pose can be practiced with or without props, though we believe the use of props can deepen your experience of savasana. Props are used if lying on the back causes any discomfort in the upper or lower back or the backs of the knees, or if you notice that your breath feels shallow or uneven.

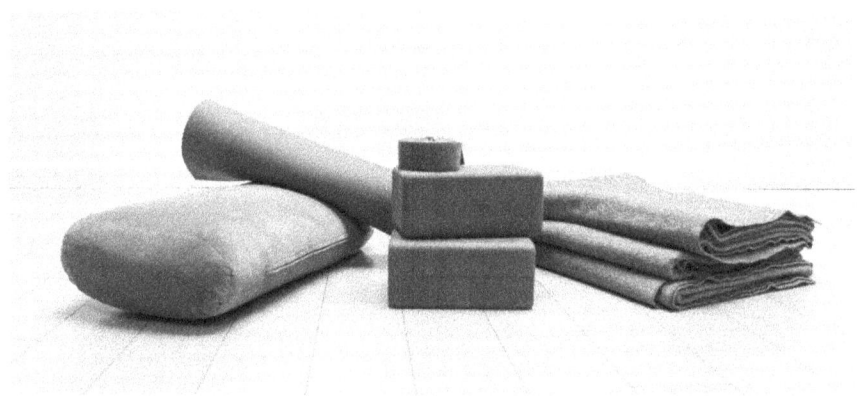

Some props that can be helpful. You can always use towels and pillows if you don't have them.

Props List

- A bolster or a few firmly rolled blankets placed under the knees. This will prevent strain on the back of the knees and reduce compression of the lower spine.

- Head support (the underside of the chin should be more or less perpendicular to the floor). Head support can be eliminated if you are able to achieve that position without it.
- An eye pillow or washcloth to cover the eyes. This will block outside light, which stimulates the brain and makes relaxation very difficult. The covering also helps to still eye movement and relaxes the eyes toward the backs of their sockets, further quieting brain activity.
- A blanket to cover the body if needed.

Instructions

1. If you are doing the pose on a yoga mat, place yourself at the center so that your heels remain padded when you lie down.
2. If you are using head support, set a blanket at one end of the mat.
3. Sit with legs extended straight out in front of you and place a rolled blanket or bolster under the knees. Place your hands behind the hips and lower yourself to the mat, first onto the elbows and forearms. Once your torso is supine, lift the pelvis slightly and use your hands to draw the skin and flesh of the buttocks toward the feet. This should lengthen, but not flatten, the lower spine. Then release the pelvis back to the mat. If discomfort arises in the low back, you may rest the calves on the seat of a chair, which is described on page 32.
4. If using head support, ensure the edge of the blanket under the head touches the top of the shoulders to support the neck. You may also roll or fold the blanket to support the curve of the neck.
5. Place your fingers at the base of the skull (on either side of the occipital

> Be as physically symmetrical as possible to calm the nervous system, but recognize that we are not inherently symmetrical. Check that the pelvis is in an anatomically neutral position— the weight of the torso is felt more on the mid-sacrum than the lumbar spine. If the lower back aches, repeat the lift and scoop of the pelvis. Place a bolster or rolled blanket under the knees for lower back support or try the version with the calves on a chair seat.

protuberance) and gently draw it away from the shoulders to lengthen the neck. Imagine the skin and flesh of the base moving up the back of the head toward the crown, while the area below the base descends down the spine and out through the tailbone.

6. If you have an eye pillow, gently close the eyes and place it evenly across them. If you prefer no weight, cover the eyes with a soft scarf instead.

7. With the arms about 45 degrees from the torso, press the elbows lightly into the mat to broaden the chest and shoulder blades evenly. Avoid over-squeezing the shoulder blades together. Turn the palms up, relax the fingers, and let the backs of the hands rest so that the fingers may curl slightly. The external rotation of the arms helps the breath flow more easily.

8. As the legs externally rotate, the skin at the back edge of the heel may catch and push toward the baby toe. Lift each foot slightly to release it. Ideally, the feet align with the hips, but some students may prefer a wider stance, especially if little or no knee support is used. If you need to widen the feet, slide them outward rather than lifting them. This movement helps the calf muscles roll outward and may relieve lower back or sacral discomfort.

9. Relax the legs, letting the feet turn out evenly. If using a bolster, ensure it is under the knee crease between the back of the thigh and the calf. If the bolster is too close to the hips, it may push the femur bones up toward the ceiling, inflate the groins, shorten the breath, and inhibit prana flow.

10. Finally, scan the body to sense whether you are symmetrical and comfortable. Adjust as needed. Even subtle imbalances can disturb the brain and lessen the effectiveness of the pose.

Balancing the body in savasana will take time and consistent practice. We use the two sides of the body in different ways in daily life. For example, the right hip may be tighter than the left. That may translate to an imbalance in the way the heels rest on the floor. Over time, you will gain awareness of any potential imbalances and adjust accordingly. Savasana will become increasingly more effective as you come closer to optimal symmetry.

What to Do in the Pose

1. Imagine the eyes softening and releasing deeply toward the backs of their sockets. Sense or envision a gentle depth at the inner corners of the eyes.

2. With the eyes closed, feel the space behind each eye and allow that space to gently widen. Notice if one side resists more than the other. Direct your awareness to that side and rest your attention there, silently encouraging the space to open and release. Often, this steady awareness helps promote letting go. Relax the eyes so that they seem to gaze under the cheekbones, or, if you prefer, toward the yoga heart behind the sternum.

3. Allow the forehead and space between the eyebrows to release from the center to the outer edges of the face. Imagine the cheekbones widening.

4. From the cheekbones, rest your awareness on the opening of each ear. Then direct your attention deeper into the ear canal. Just as one eye may hold more tension, so too can the inner ears. Notice which side feels more spacious and which feels compressed. Rest your awareness on the smaller or tighter side, gently encouraging it to let go. With each exhalation, imagine tension draining from the ears.

5. Feel for any holding in the hinges of the jaw, just in front of the ears. Release all effort there so completely that you cannot tell whether the upper and lower teeth are touching or not.

6. Soften and widen the lips until you are unsure whether they are touching or not.

7. Visualize the gums and the palate as free of tension, inviting these tissues to broaden and soften.

8. Sense the midline of the tongue, running from its tip to its base in the throat. Let the base of the tongue be wide, with its tip lightly resting on the roof of the mouth behind the front teeth. In a supine position, if the tongue falls to the bottom of the mouth, it may drop toward the throat and briefly impede the breath.

9. Allow or imagine the back of the throat to gently widen and soften.

10. Observe the movement of the breath as it brushes against the inner nostrils. At first, the inhalation may seem to touch different areas—for example, the upper nostril on the right, the lower on the left. Guide the inhalation so that it touches evenly along the sides of the septum, keeping the nostrils soft. Then sense the exhalation flowing toward the outer edges of the nostrils.

11. Imagine the torso as an empty, flexible vessel. Envision removing the organs so that you are left with a spacious "pot." Invite the inhalation to fill this pot in every direction—vertically, horizontally, and circumferentially. With the exhalation, feel the release of all sides of the torso drawing inward toward a central line from the center of the pelvic floor, the perineum, to the crown of the head.

12. Observe the area from the sitting bones to the collarbones. As the inhalation begins, imagine it first touching the perineum. Like filling a glass of water from bottom to top, sense the pelvic floor widening, the sitting bones moving slightly apart, and the tailbone lengthening away from the pubic bone.

13. As the exhalation leaves, brushing the outer nostrils, imagine it first departing from the perineum. Sense the sitting bones gently drawing toward each other and the tailbone moving slightly toward the pubic bone.

14. Bring your awareness to the spine. Imagine the muscles that run along both sides softening and widening outward from the center.

15. Observe the lungs and the inner frame of the rib cage. Notice that each lung expands with the inhalation, though not always evenly. Invite the more resistant lung to fill more fully on the inhale. As you exhale, visualize tension releasing from that side.

16. Allow the skin across the sternum to soften and spread. Sense the inside edge of the sternum widening in all directions. Let the collarbones extend outward from the sternum toward the tops of the shoulders, then imagine them lifting and rolling gently over the shoulders.

17. As you settle into this stillness, feel the body gently sinking into the earth. Sense the weight of the body releasing downward. Imagine the back of the body spreading outward in all directions, like a drop of water meeting the ground. Allow yourself to fully relax, surrendering into connection with the earth beneath you. As the body releases into stillness, the mind will naturally follow.

The breath can be the bridge between the conscious and the unconscious. Whether the bridge is open depends on a balance of optimal conditions and grace.

When we can quiet our thoughts and simply become a witness to the breath, more may be revealed. It is possible that you come to recognize your true nature is love and kindness and that you are connected to everything.

Stay in savasana for a minimum of 10–15 minutes and up to 60 minutes, if possible. However, adjust the time to your needs. When we asked our teacher Ramanand Patel what happens if a person doesn't have an hour for savasana, he advised doing the pose for 59 minutes.

Exiting the Pose

Roll gently to one side, using your top arm to push you up to a seated position. Move slowly, and sit quietly for a few moments in any seated position, noticing how you feel. This is a minimal instruction for exiting; chapter 6 offers more detailed guidance on leaving the pose with awareness.

Modifications

- Place a small support under your Achilles tendons if you have discomfort from the heels resting on the floor.
- Cover yourself with a blanket if you have a tendency to feel cold.

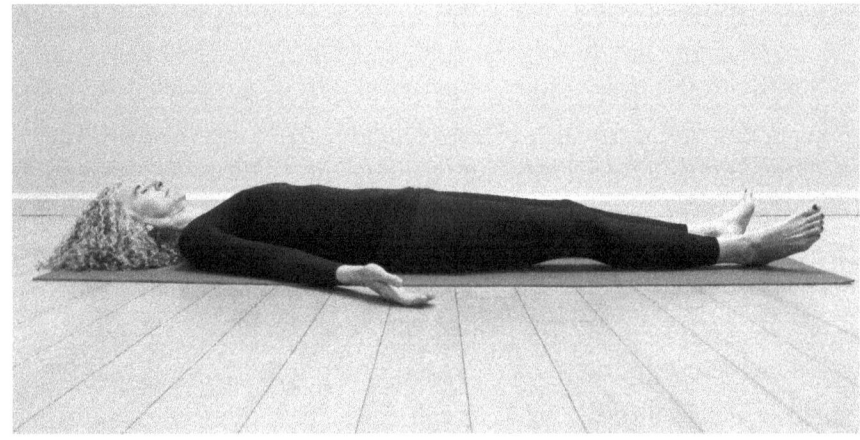

FIGURE 1: Unsupported savasana, side view

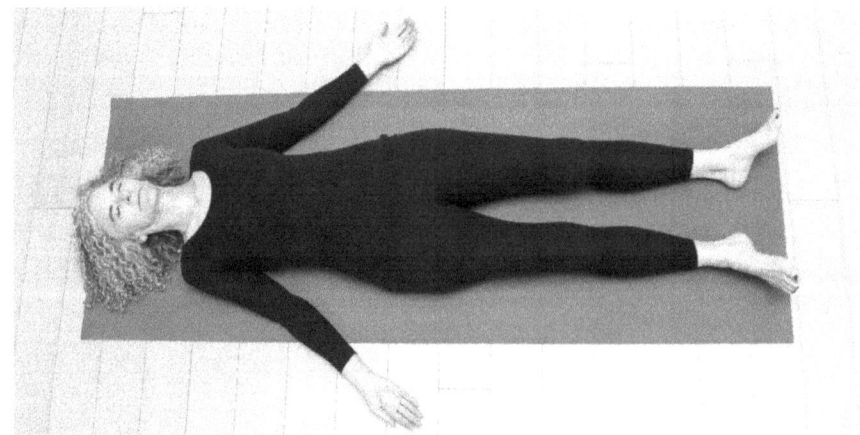

FIGURE 2: View from above. Feet are hip width apart and the arms form equal angles relative to the the torso.

Savasana: Getting in, Getting out 19

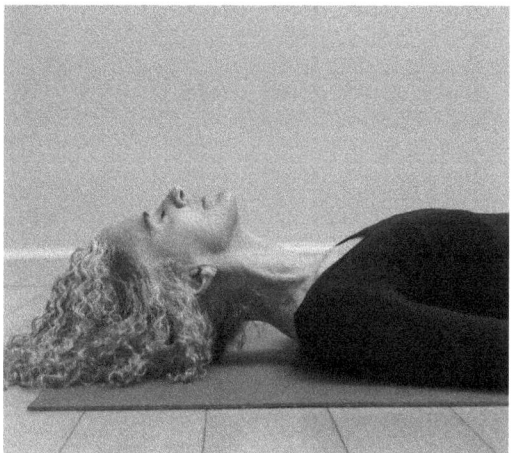
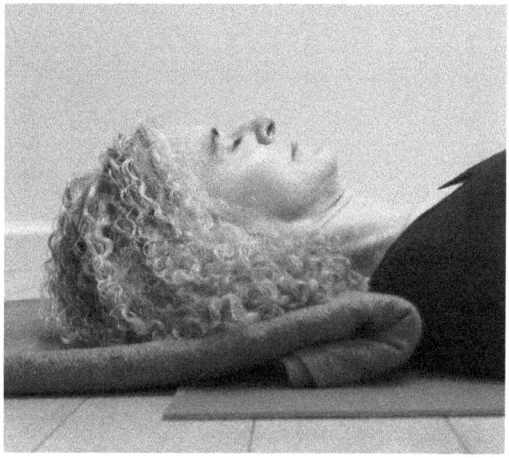

FIGURES 3A AND 3B: (*above*) The cervical curve is too deep, tightening the neck muscles and pushing the chin up and back. A blanket support is needed, rolled just deep enough to bring the cervical spine back to normal.

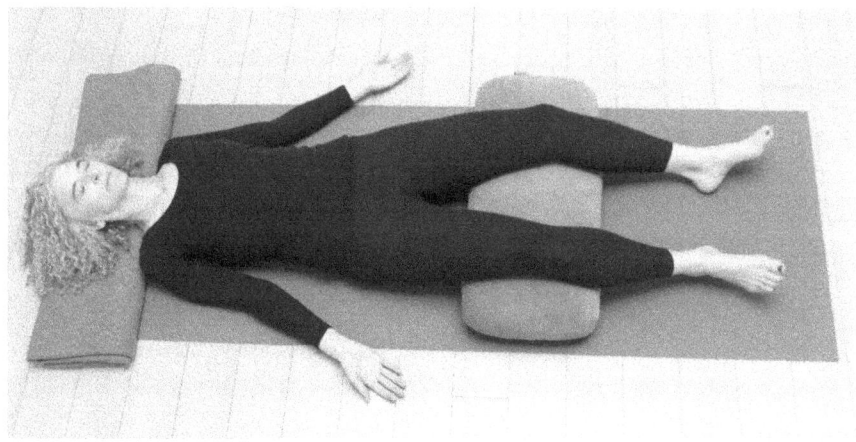

FIGURE 4: Savasana with supports, a bolster for the knees and a folded blanket for the neck.

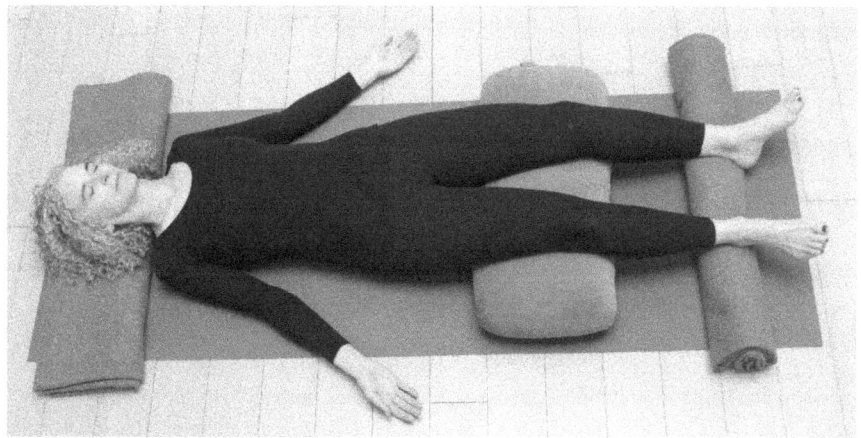

FIGURE 5: Supported savasana, using the supports illustrated in figure 4, but adding a rolled blanket for the ankles.

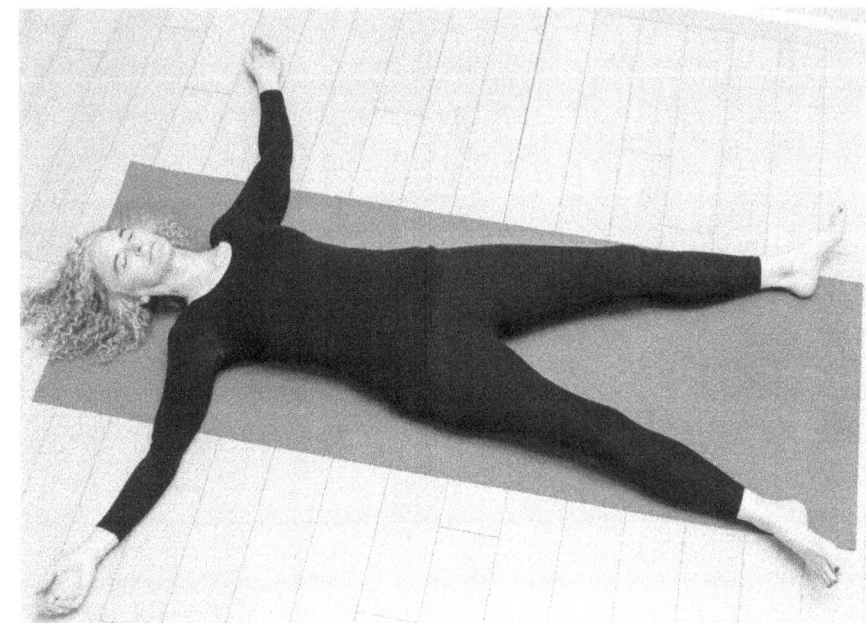

FIGURE 6: What *not* to do in savasana. Legs are too wide, arms are too high, which affects the shoulders, and the head is tilted, out of alignment with the spine.

- Tuck the blanket under the outside edge of your legs to keep them more internally rotated if you have sacroiliac discomfort. Alternatively, put a yoga strap around the thighs so they are more internally rotated.

Sometimes a student simply collapses into a version of savasana that our teacher Ramanand jokingly calls "dead cowboy," evoking the image of those motionless heroes (or villains) from old spaghetti westerns. This position, however, is far from ideal for receiving the full benefits of a well-aligned and, when needed, supported pose.

Savasana with Weight on the Thighs

Overview

This variation builds upon the supported savasana setup but introduces weight across the upper thighs to deepen the breath and release tension in the hip flexors. The gentle downward pressure lengthens the psoas muscles and encourages the breath to move more fully into the lower torso. A bolster, folded blankets, or sandbags can be used, and for students who need greater intensity, a plate weight of up to 30 pounds is an option. Interestingly, many practitioners notice that their lungs expand more with added weight, lengthening the inhale. Placing weight asymmetrically with more weight on the tighter quadricep can help create more balance and symmetry in the breath.

Props List

- Two or three blankets (plus a fourth if you don't have a bolster)
- A bolster or two rolled blankets placed under the knees (this support is essential for the variation)
- One folded blanket or an extra mat to spread across the thighs, creating a base for the weights
- Optional blanket to cover the body for warmth
- Two yoga sandbags (8–10 pounds each) or a plate weight (20–30 pounds)
- Note: If using a plate weight, place an extra yoga mat over the thighs to prevent slipping and keep a block nearby to support the plate at a low height for easier transfer.
- Optional yoga strap if you have any history of sacral instability

Instructions

1. Begin by setting up your savasana as described in Classic Supine Savasana, but keep your chosen weight close at hand before reclining. If you are using sandbags, place one on each side of your mat. If you are working with a plate weight, set it securely on a block at a low height next to your thighs so you can easily slide it onto your body once reclined.

2. Ideally, another person can place the weights for you. If you are practicing alone, here are a few safe approaches:

   - Sandbags: Position them across your upper thighs before lying down. Place each sandbag about 1–2 inches below the hip crease, with slightly more weight resting toward the outer thigh to encourage the legs to roll outward. Take care: Once you lie back, adjusting the buttocks flesh may be more challenging with the bags in place, and they can slide if not secure.

   - Plate: Do not attempt to position the plate until you are reclined. Once lying back, drag the plate from the block onto the folded blanket or extra mat across your thighs, adjusting its position so the weight is evenly supported.

3. Once the weight is in place, allow your body to respond to the sensation. Notice the subtle shifts in your breathing. The weight helps guide the diaphragm downward and creates more space for the lower lungs to expand.

Exiting the Pose

1. If you are practicing alone, remove the weights before making any larger movements:

   - Sandbags: Slide one bag at a time off to the side, allowing it to rest on the floor. Move slowly to avoid strain.

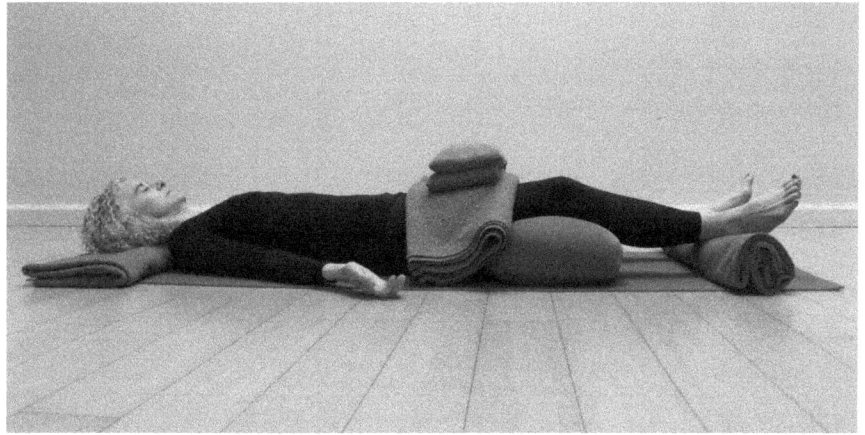

FIGURE 7: Supported savasana, side view, using the same setup as in (5), but this time with two 10-pound sandbags laid across the top of the thighs, padded by a blanket.

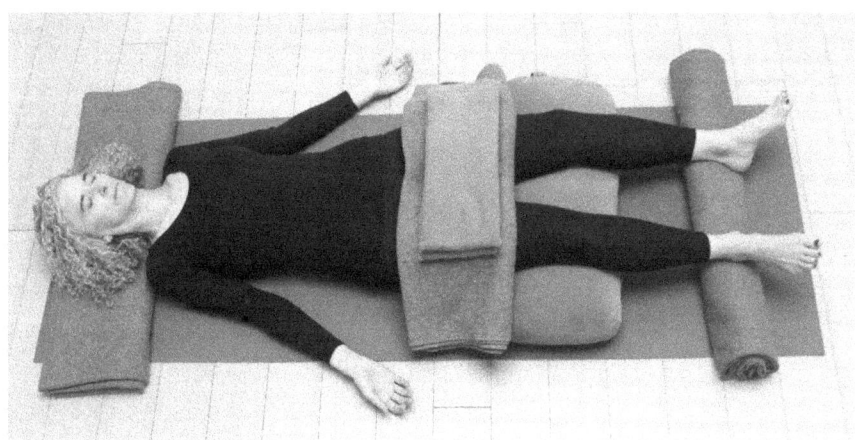

FIGURE 8: Supported savasana with weight, view from above.

- Plate: Carefully drag the plate from your thighs back onto the supporting block. Ensure it is secure before moving further.

2. Once the weights are removed, pause for a few breaths to notice how the body feels without them.

3. Roll gently to one side, using your arms to help you transition to a seated position. Move slowly, as the body may feel especially heavy and grounded after this practice.

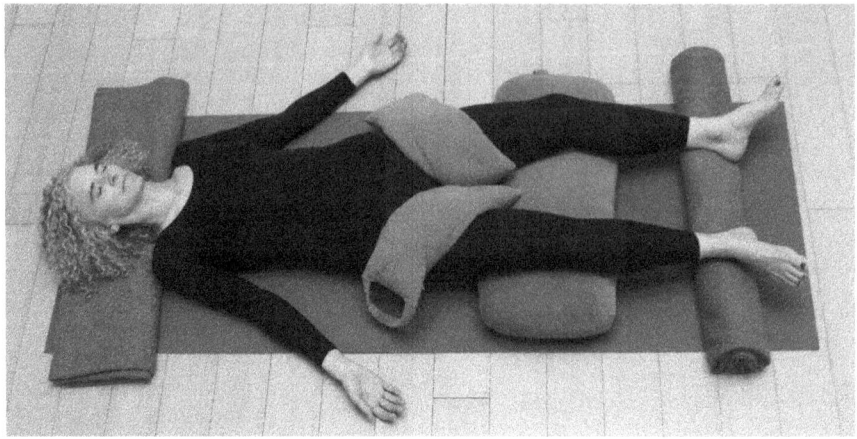

FIGURE 9: The supported setup as in (8) with the sandbags this time laid across the front groins, parallel to the lines of the hip crease.

Modifications

If you have a history of sacral pain or instability, place a looped belt around the mid-thighs before putting weight on the thigh bones. This helps prevent excessive external rotation of the femurs that can occur under load.

With sandbags, experiment with weight distribution:

- Shift more sand toward the outer thigh to encourage greater external rotation.
- Shift more sand inward for less rotation, which can be important for those with sacral or lower back discomfort.
- If you need asymmetrical breath work, stack the sandbags or adjust them so one side of the body receives more pressure, helping the breath expand more evenly between the lungs.

If using a plate weight, ensure the blanket or mat beneath it fully prevents slipping, and always move the weight with care.

This variation combines grounding pressure with supported rest, making it a powerful way to release the deep hip flexors, balance the breath, and quiet the nervous system.

Savasana with Weight on the Heads of the Humeri

Overview

This variation builds on the standard savasana setup and is designed to gently open the chest and shoulders by directing weight into the heads of the humerus bones, where the upper arm bones meet the shoulder sockets. The grounding pressure encourages the shoulders to release downward, broadens the collarbones, and helps soften tension through the upper back and chest.

> This variation can be challenging to set up alone. Because precise placement is key, it's best practiced with the help of a teacher, partner, or friend. For safety and alignment, have another person position the sandbags whenever possible. If you're practicing solo, move slowly and proceed with care.

Props List

- Standard props for savasana (bolster or blanket support under knees, head and neck support if needed, eye pillow, blanket for warmth)
- Two yoga sandbags (approximately 10 pounds each)
- Optional: a partner or assistant to help place the sandbags

Instructions

1. Begin in your regular savasana position. Place support under the knees or calves and head support if needed, making sure the blanket is also supporting the neck.

2. Before placing the sandbags, shift the sand toward one of the short ends of each bag. Concentrating the weight at one end allows for more targeted placement at the shoulder joint.

3. With the help of a partner (or as carefully as possible if alone), position each sandbag with the heavier end a few inches above the armpit crease, directly over the head of the humerus. The bag should rest in the hollow where the upper arm meets the shoulder socket.

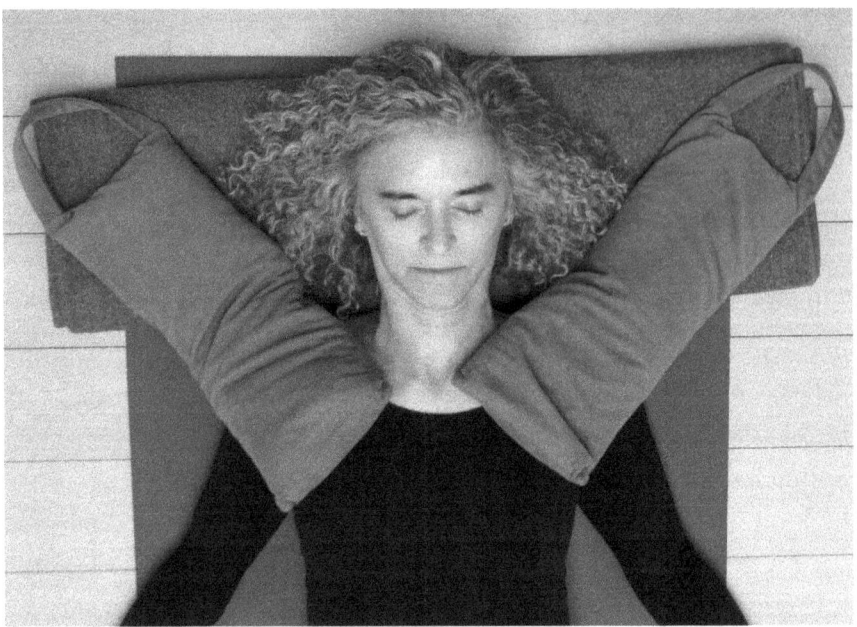

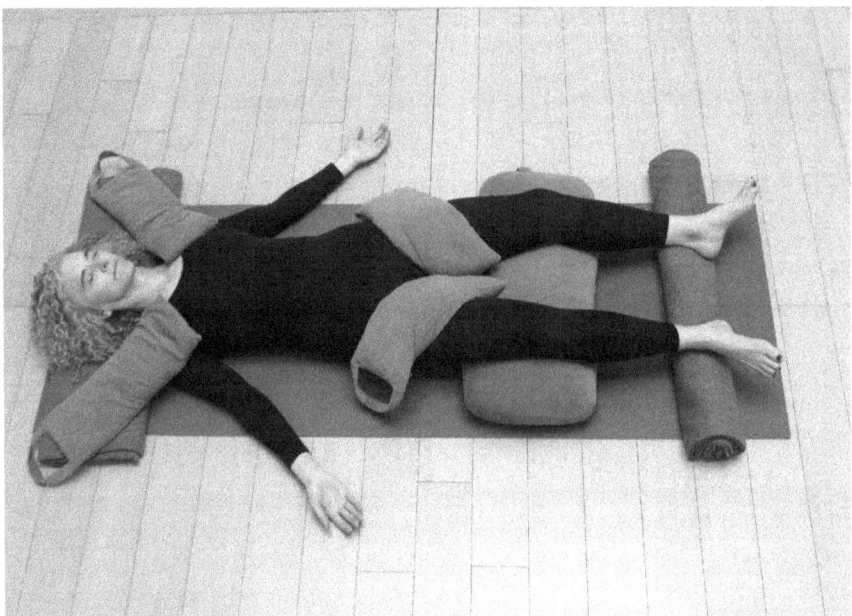

FIGURES 10A AND 10B: Sandbags to help release the shoulders. Notice that they are placed so that they are at equal angles to the sides of the neck and weigh equally on the shoulders. Feel the shoulders drop down and out to the sides. Feedback from the sandbags may bring more awareness of differences between the shoulders with one humerus being higher toward the ceiling than the other.

Because the sand will naturally slide toward the floor, gently press the sand back toward the body so the heaviest part of the bag remains in contact with the shoulder joint.

4. Settle and soften: Once the bags are in place, close your eyes and bring awareness to the sensations in the shoulders and chest.

    - Feel the shoulders drop down and out to the sides. Feedback from the sandbags may bring more awareness of differences between the shoulders with one humerus lifted higher toward the ceiling than the other. There is more tightness in that side of the chest. Just by thinking about it, try to allow the holding and tension on that side to relax and lengthen.
    - Allow or imagine the collarbones broadening.
    - Allow or imagine the arms growing longer and the upper arm bones releasing toward the floor.

5. Remain in this variation for 5–15 minutes, letting the weight on the heads of the humeri invite openness across the chest and the release of habitual tension in the shoulders.

Exiting the Pose

1. If working with a partner, ask them to carefully lift the sandbags off your shoulders before you begin moving.
2. If practicing alone, bend elbows slightly, one at a time, and gently guide the bag on that shoulder off to the side of the body, moving slowly to avoid strain.
3. Once the weights are removed, pause for several breaths to sense the rebound effect in the shoulders and chest.
4. When ready, roll to one side and press up slowly to a seated position.

This variation offers a deep yet supported chest opening, ideal for countering slouched posture, releasing shoulder tightness, and cultivating a sense of spaciousness in the upper body.

Savasana with Weight on the Forehead

Overview

This variation builds upon the foundational savasana instructions. As we've seen with using weight on the thighs, or shoulders, applying steady pressure to a specific area can stimulate the parasympathetic nervous system and invite deeper relaxation. While weight on the forehead may sound unusual—or even like the invention of an overzealous yoga teacher—many students find it profoundly calming. Of course, it won't resonate with everyone, but for some, it provides a unique gateway to stillness and quiet.

Props List

- Two yoga blocks
- One sandbag (approximately 10 pounds) or another soft, stable weight
- One small rolled towel

Instructions

1. Place the rolled towel under the cervical spine to support the natural curve of the neck. It should feel supportive but not so thick that it lifts the head.
2. Place two blocks lengthwise on the floor just above the crown of the head. Stand them on their sides (middle height) so they are broad, stable, and touching one another. The ends should lightly touch or come very close to the crown of the head.
3. Ideally, have someone else place the sandbag for accuracy. If practicing alone, move slowly and carefully.
    - Place the sandbag lengthwise, on and parallel to the blocks, with any straps at the far end, away from the head.
    - Distribute the weight so that half rests on the blocks and half rests gently across the forehead.

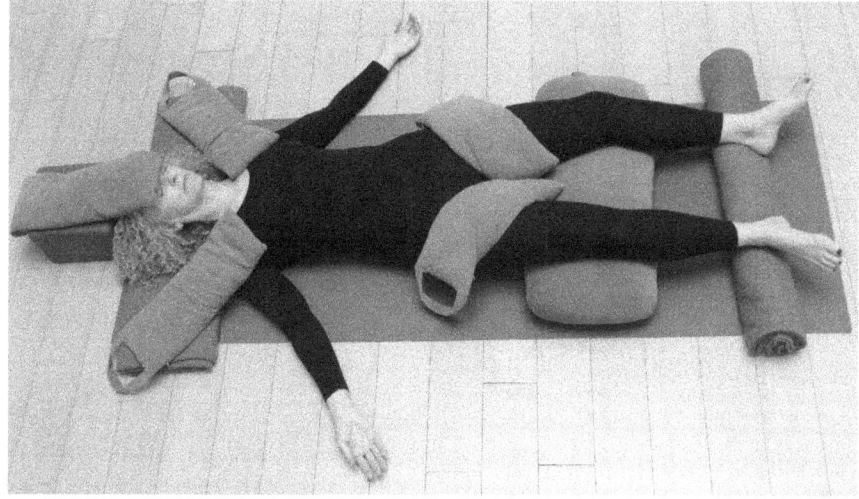

FIGURE 11A: Sandbag on the forehead. Imagine the brain gently shrinking, drawing inward toward its center.

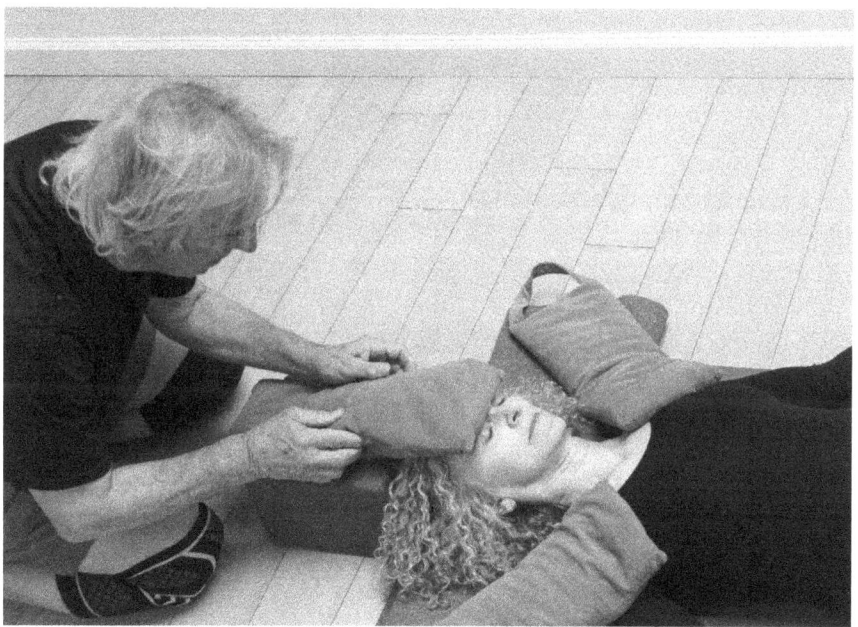

FIGURE 11B: Adjusting the sandbag on the forehead. Note the weight of the bag is balanced on two blocks and the forehead. Make sure the sandbag is gently pushing the forehead skin toward the nose.

- Ensure the bag does not press on the eyes.

4. If the weight pulls the skin of the forehead upward, slide your fingertips under the edge of the bag and gently draw the skin downward toward the bridge of the nose, then outward toward the temples. This softens the frontalis muscle (the forehead muscle linked with expressive movement and tension), signaling the brain to release and settle.

5. With the weight in place, invite a subtle inward and downward sensation in the head:

    - Imagine the brain gently shrinking, drawing inward toward its center.
    - Imagine the brain gently sinking, settling back toward the base of the skull (the occiput).

6. Remain for 5–10 minutes, or longer if comfortable, allowing the steady pressure and stillness to quiet the nervous system and encourage deep relaxation.

Exiting the Pose

To exit the pose, bend the knees to place the feet on the floor. Then, reach overhead to lift the weight off of the forehead. Before rolling to your side, notice how you feel. Does the mind feel quiet? After rolling to one side, use your top hand pushing into the floor to help you come up to any seated position. Sit quietly for a few breaths.

Modifications

Optional: The Glabella Release

The glabella, Latin for "smooth," is the small area between the eyebrows. Yogic traditions recognize this point as the seat of the sixth chakra, the *ajna* or "command wheel."

For this variation, you'll need:

- A yoga block (firm foam, cork, or bamboo preferred)

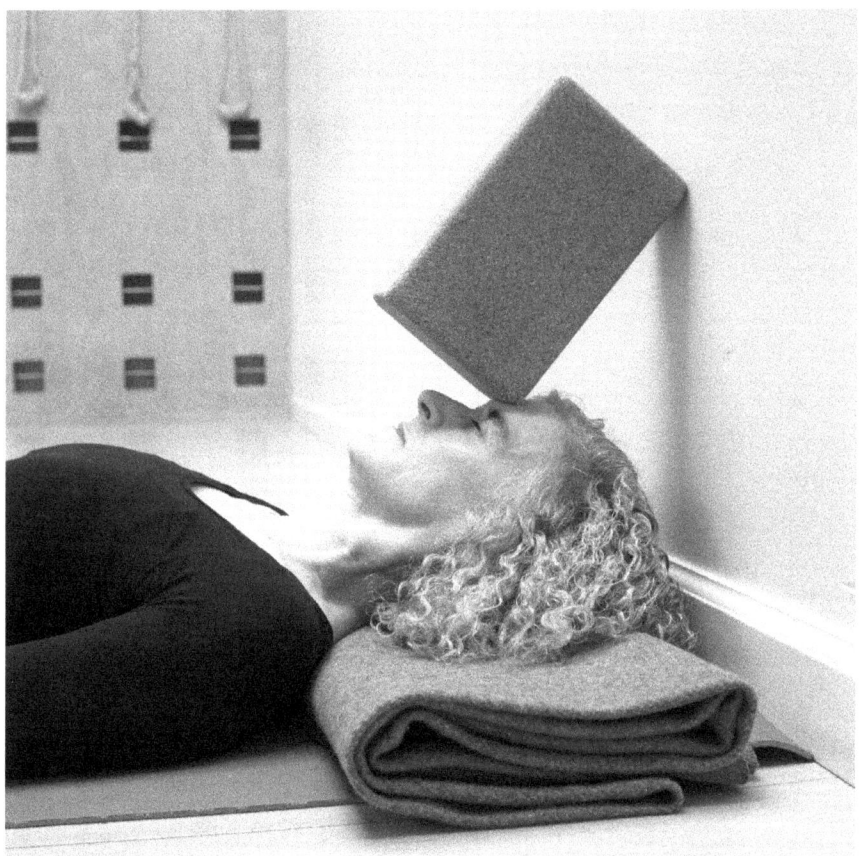

FIGURE 12: The "glabella block," angled between a wall and the bridge of the nose (glabella). Notice the head and neck are comfortably supported on a folded blanket.

- A small sticky-mat square (about 3 inches across) for padding
- A wall for support

How to Practice the Glabella Release

1. Lie on your back with the crown of the head about 3–4 inches from the wall (roughly the width of a block). Legs may rest over a bolster or with knees bent, feet on the floor.

2. Position the block lengthwise, one short edge against the wall and the opposite edge resting just above the glabella. Note this works better with a cork block. If using a foam block, you may want to have a small piece of yoga mat between the corner of the block and the forehead.

3. Slowly let the block slide down until it settles into place against the glabella, gently drawing the skin downward toward the nose.
4. Rest quietly for a few minutes, noticing any subtle effects.

This practice may not appeal to everyone, and the effects may be very subtle at first. Try it for three or four short sessions, and see what reveals itself.

This forehead variation of savasana, along with the optional glabella release, provides a unique way to calm the mind, soften habitual forehead tension, and deepen the body's capacity for stillness.

Supported Savasana with Chair

Overview

This restorative variation of savasana is particularly supportive for students who experience discomfort in the lower back, tightness in the hip flexors, or difficulty fully releasing into the traditional posture. By resting the lower legs on a chair, the thighs can gently release into the hip sockets, which in turn eases tension in the lumbar spine. The position also promotes healthy blood flow and provides a deeply grounding experience, making it especially beneficial for those who struggle to find ease and relaxation when lying flat on the floor.

Props List

- One sturdy chair (folding or dining style with no wheels, to prevent slipping)
- A folded blanket on the chair seat (optional, for added cushioning, especially important if using a metal chair)
- A rolled towel or small bolster under the ankles (optional, for extra comfort)
- Standard savasana props: head support such as a folded blanket, an eye cover to reduce light and quiet the senses, and an additional blanket for warmth

Savasana: Getting in, Getting out 33

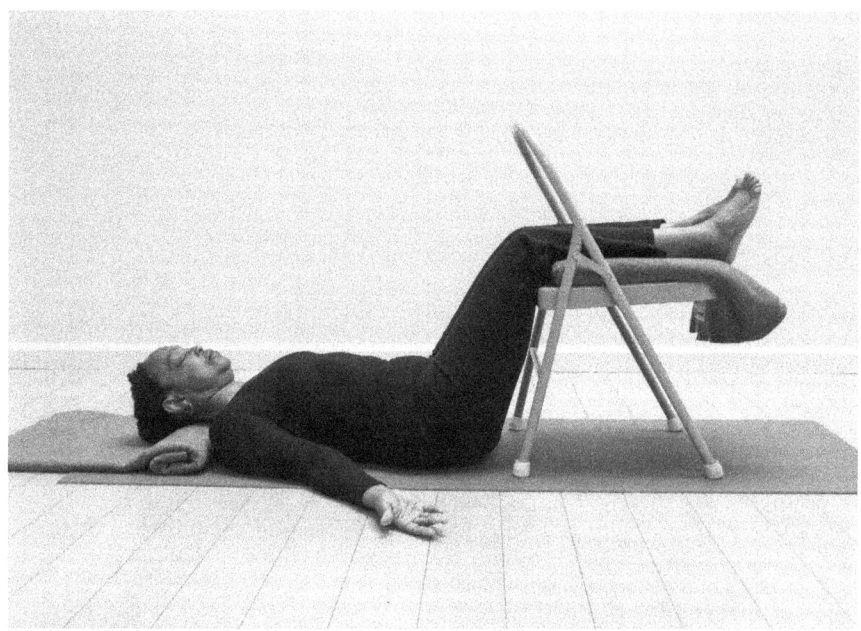

FIGURE 13: Side view of savasana with legs supported on a chair. Notice the neck support and the blanket padding the chair seat.

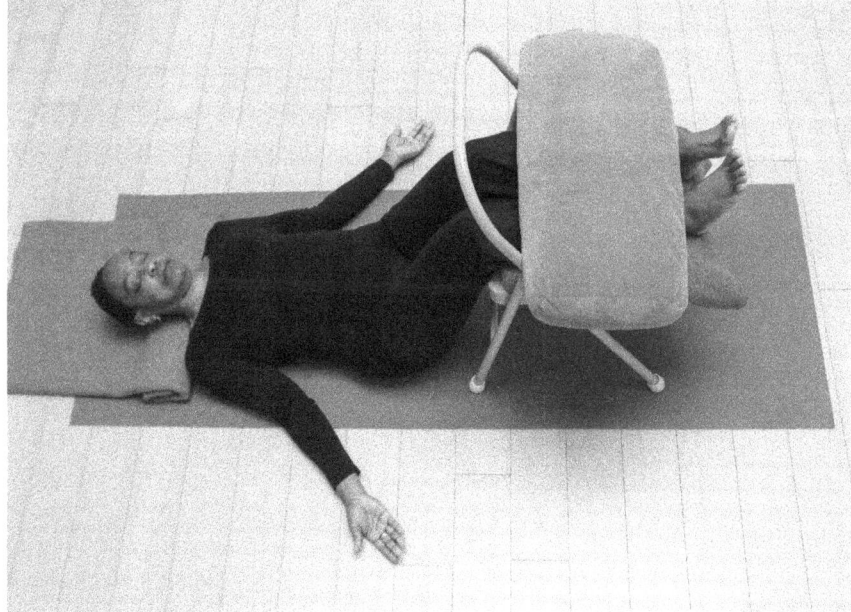

FIGURE 14: Top view of savasana with a bolster weight across the shins.

Instructions

1. Place your chair securely at the end of your yoga mat with the seat facing you. Positioning it on the mat helps prevent slipping when weight is applied.

    If you're using a traditional metal folding chair, note that the seat tilts slightly downward toward the back. For this reason, it may be more comfortable and supportive to turn the chair so that the backrest faces you. This way, the front edge of the seat slopes slightly up and away from your calves, creating a more favorable angle for the legs.

2. Sit down in front of the chair, close to its base, and then slowly roll onto your back. As you do so, move the pelvis toward the chair and lift your legs onto the seat, until the backs of your knees rest comfortably at the edge of the chair seat. Ideally, your knees should bend to about 90 degrees with the calves fully supported by the seat.

3. If you find that the chair feels too high or too low for your body proportions, make adjustments: add a folded blanket on the chair seat to raise the legs, or place a folded blanket beneath the pelvis or upper back to raise your torso. These small changes ensure that the position feels balanced and supportive.

4. If you notice pressure building behind the ankles, slide a rolled towel or small blanket under them so the feet and ankles can soften without strain.

5. Take a moment to check your pelvis: the weight should be centered on the sacrum, rather than tipping the lower back into an exaggerated arch away from the ground. A neutral pelvis creates a more even release throughout the spine.

6. From here, set yourself up as you would in traditional savasana:

    - Gently lengthen the buttocks flesh down toward the heels, encouraging space in the lower back.

- Place supportive padding under the head and neck if the chin tips upward or if you feel strain.
- Cover the eyes with a soft cloth or eye pillow to invite the gaze inward and calm the mind.
- If the body cools easily, drape a blanket over yourself for warmth and comfort.
- Extend the arms slightly away from the torso, about 45 degrees, with palms turned upward in a gesture of openness.

7. Once settled, allow your breath to become soft and effortless. Each exhale can invite the body to release more deeply into the support beneath you. Stay here for 10–20 minutes, letting the nervous system reset and the body rest completely.

Exiting the Pose

Roll gently to one side, using your top arm to push you up to a seated position. Move slowly, and sit for a few moments in any seated position noticing how you feel.

Modifications

- If the legs rolling outward causes discomfort, place a yoga strap around the thighs to encourage alignment of the thighs in line with the hips and to prevent strain.
- For an added sense of grounding, place a bolster lengthwise across the shins. A sandbag on top of the bolster can increase the feeling of being anchored and help encourage parasympathetic relaxation.
- If the chair edge presses uncomfortably into the backs of the knees, place a folded blanket along the edge to soften the contact and prevent compression.

This supported variation of savasana provides a safe, nurturing way to rest the body and calm the mind, making it an excellent choice for restorative practices, recovery days, or any time you wish to experience deep release without effort.

Reclining Bound Angle Pose (Supta Baddha Konasana)

Overview

While supta baddha konasana is not traditionally considered a form of savasana, it can serve as a restorative alternative. This pose opens the hips and chest, provides gentle traction to the lower back, encourages relaxation of the sacral ligaments and releases the psoas. It requires more setup and props than traditional savasana, but for those who invest the time, it can be deeply restorative.

Props List

- One bolster
- Three blankets
- Two blocks
- One yoga strap, fastened into a large loop
- Optional: sandbags for added grounding
- Optional: yoga eye pillow or cloth to cover the eyes

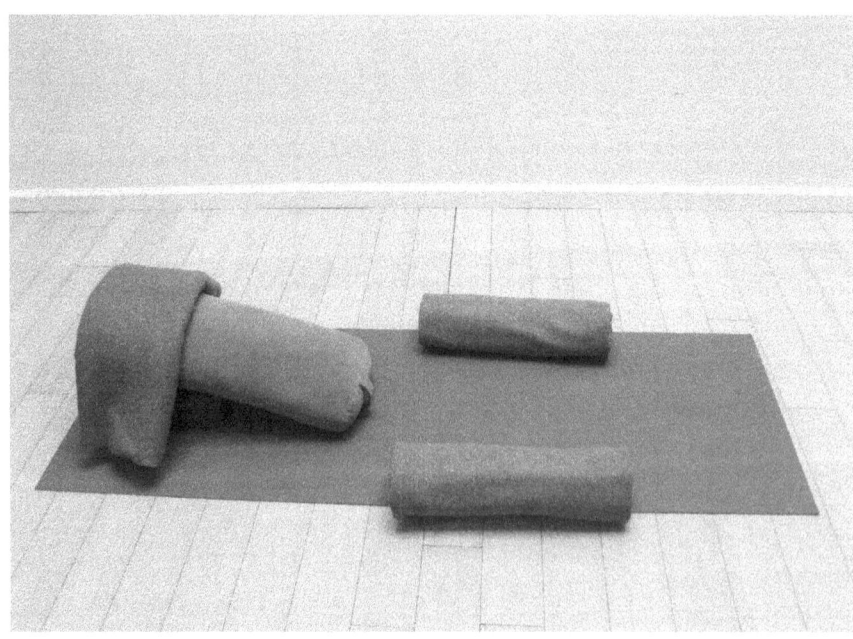

FIGURE 15: Prop setup for savasana with legs in reclining bound angle pose (supta baddha konasana). The bolster is angled on two blocks, one low and the other medium height.

Instructions

1. Place the bolster lengthwise at the back of the mat. Prop the far end with one low block and one medium block to create a gentle slant. Fold a blanket on top of the bolster to cushion the head and neck.
2. Sit facing away from the bolster in bound angle pose, leaving 2–3 inches between your buttocks and the front edge of the bolster.
3. Place rolled blankets under the outer thighs as close to the hips as possible. Adjust the thickness to reduce any inner thigh stretch when reclining.
4. Loop the strap behind the torso down across the sacrum above the tailbone. Pass it over the inner thighs and around the outer edges of the feet. Pull taut, ensuring it stays low on the sacrum and does not ride up onto the lumbar spine.
5. Lie back onto the bolster. Optionally, lift the pelvis slightly and draw the buttocks flesh away from the lower back to lengthen the lumbar area.
6. Focus on slow, deep breaths for 5–20 minutes (longer if comfortable), noticing the expansion of the chest and the release through the hips and lower back.

Exiting the Pose

To exit the pose, place hands under the thighs and bring knees together. Remove feet from the strap. Bend knees, roll to one side, and press up to seated using the hands.

Modifications

- Place an eye pillow or cloth over the eyes to reduce visual stimulation and deepen relaxation.
- Ensure you are seated in front of the bolster with a few inches between you and the bolster. If the lower back feels

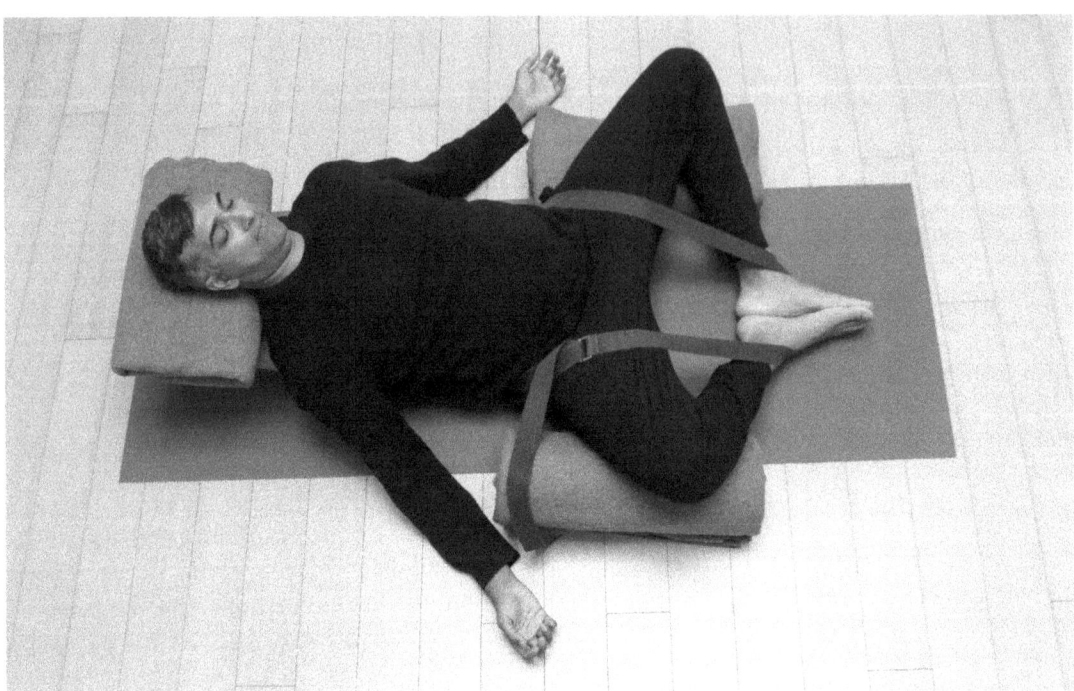

FIGURE 16: (*above*) Savasana in reclining bound angle pose. Notice the yoga belt around the back pelvis, over the inner thighs, and around the outer feet.

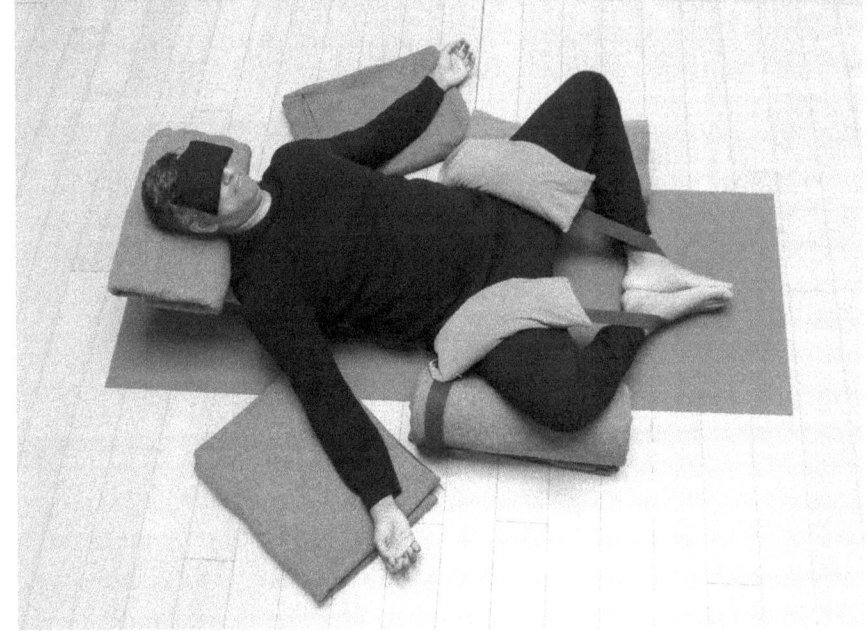

FIGURE 17: Supta baddha konasana with eye pillow and sandbags placed on the tops of the thighs, showing proper support underneath the thighs with rolled blankets.

uncomfortable, fold a blanket or two the long skinny way to place on top of the bolster to make it higher.

- While the strap greatly enhances benefits by lengthening the lower back, stabilizing the sacrum, and gently holding the feet together, the pose can be practiced without it.
- Use extra folded blankets or blocks under the forearms, palms up, or rest the hands on the belly for additional comfort.
- For grounding, place sandbags on the tops of the thighs, ensuring proper support underneath with bolsters or blocks.

Prone Savasana or Sea-Monster Pose (Makrasana)

Overview

Makrasana, or sea-monster pose, is a face-down variation of savasana that promotes awareness along the back of the body and encourages the pratyahara state—withdrawal of the senses—by having the head face down. This posture helps lengthen and release the psoas muscles and provides a unique counterbalance to the usual supine resting poses.

Props List

- One firm bolster (or blankets/towels folded into a firm, skinny rectangle)
- Three or more blankets, depending on available props

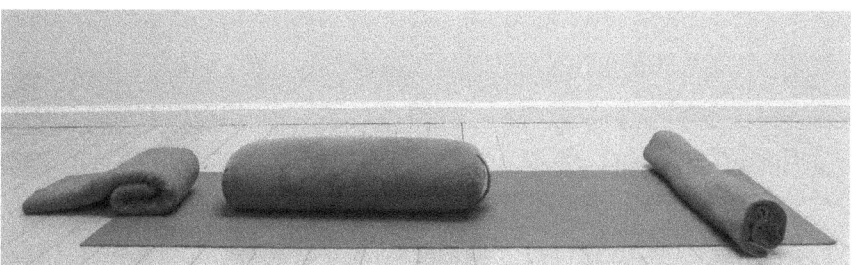

Prop setup for face-down prone savasana.

Instructions

1. Place the bolster lengthwise on the mat. Fold one blanket from a rectangle into a skinny rectangle and then fold from the short end three times, creating a height nearly equal to the bolster. Position it at one end of the bolster about 6–8 inches from the edge to support the forehead.
2. Roll a second blanket into a skinny rectangle for the ankles to rest on. This reduces pressure on the front of the knees.
3. Begin kneeling at the end of the mat near the ankle support. Place the tops of your ankles on the roll so that your feet hang off. Using your hands for support, lower your torso onto the bolster facing down, aligning the middle of your sternum with the top edge of the bolster.
4. Ensure the folded blanket under your forehead allows space for your nose, mouth, and throat, keeping the airway free.
5. Place the arms in a cactus shape, with upper arms aligned with the armpits and hands facing down roughly at head height.
6. Remain in the pose for 5–15 minutes, or longer if comfortable, noticing the breath moving along each side of the spine and the gentle release in the psoas.

Exiting the Pose

Slide your hands near chest level, push back into child's pose, resting your forehead on the bolster for a few breaths, then slowly rise to a seated position.

Modifications

- If you experience lower back discomfort, place a small towel or skinny folded blanket between the pubic bone and navel on the bolster.
- For larger or sensitive breasts, place a folded blanket lengthwise along the bolster about one-third of the way down from the head, creating a negative space to reduce pressure.

Savasana: Getting in, Getting out   41

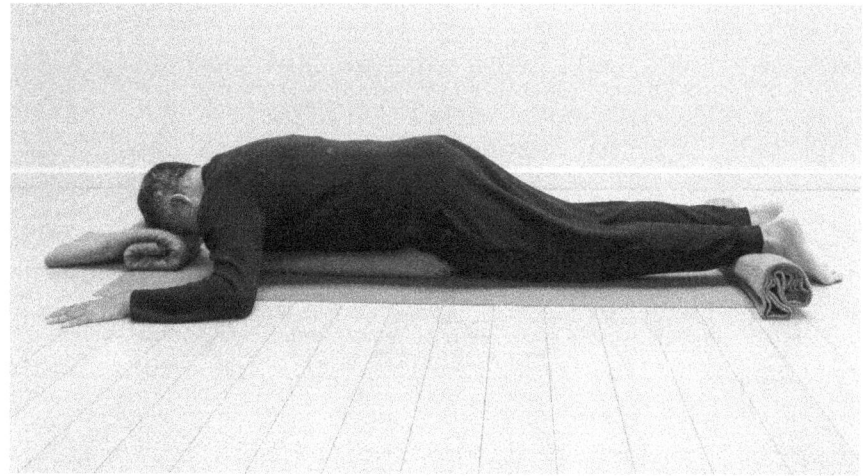

FIGURE 18: Side view of face-down savasana. The torso is resting on a lengthwise bolster, the forehead on a folded blanket, and the ankles on a blanket roll. Notice the "cactus" position of the arms.

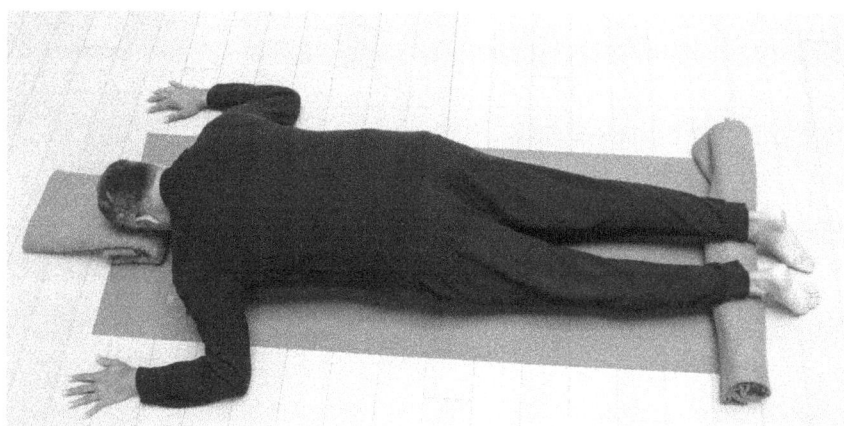

FIGURE 19: Face-down savasana as shown from above.

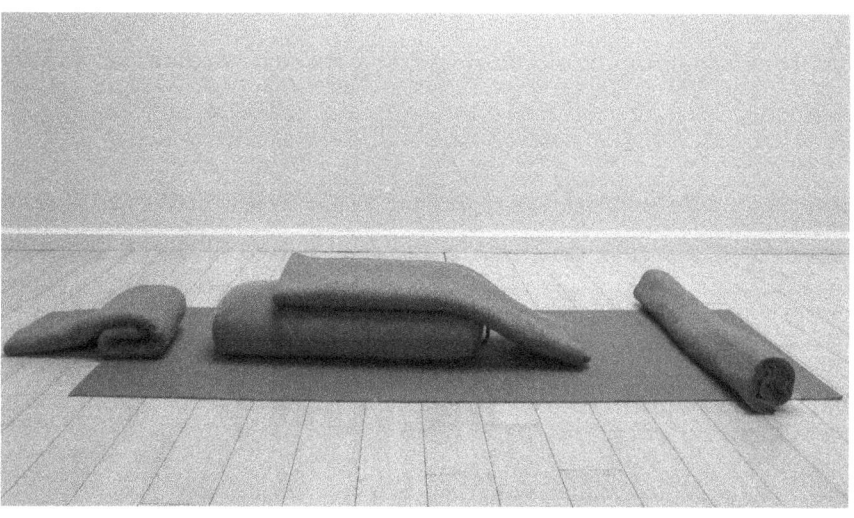

FIGURE 20: Prop setup for prone savasana with extra support if the breasts are large or sensitive when face down.

Makrasana provides a restorative, sensory-withdrawal experience that emphasizes back awareness, breath, and gentle psoas release, offering a complementary alternative to supine savasana variations.

Side-Lying Savasana (Parsva Savasana)

Overview

Side-lying savasana is an excellent option for those who find lying flat on the back uncomfortable or contraindicated, such as during pregnancy, post-surgery, or with certain spinal conditions. Parsva savasana is deeply calming and grounding, supports blood flow, eases lower back pressure, and fosters a sense of emotional safety. Pregnant practitioners are traditionally advised to lie on the left side to avoid compressing the inferior vena cava, a major vein returning blood to the heart. The goal, as with all savasana variations, is to feel fully supported and still.

Props List

- One or two firm blankets or a bolster to place between the knees
- One small pillow or folded blanket for head support
- Optional blanket for the upper arm or under the waist for added comfort
- Eye pillow or light cloth to cover the eyes
- Optional blanket to cover the body for warmth

Instructions

1. Position your mat lengthwise near a wall for additional support or grounding if desired.
2. Gently lie down on your right or left side, aligning the spine from head to tailbone.

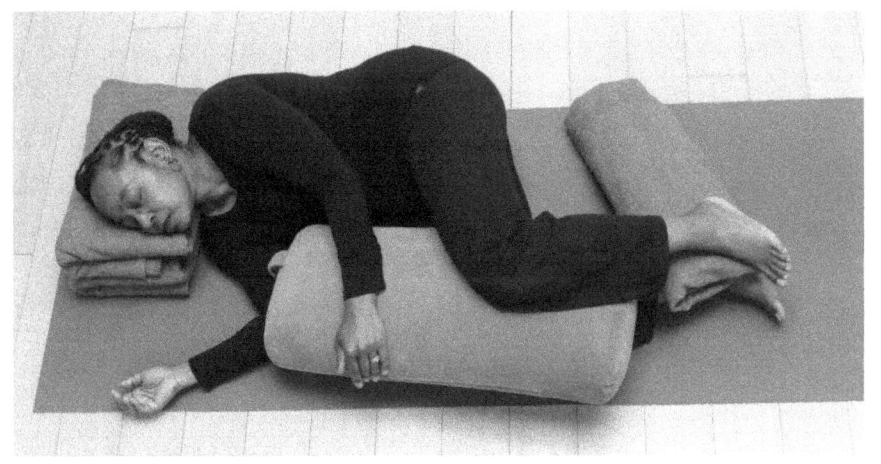

FIGURE 21: Side-lying savasana. Notice the bolster between the legs, which also serves to support the upper arm, and the folded blanket between the ankles.

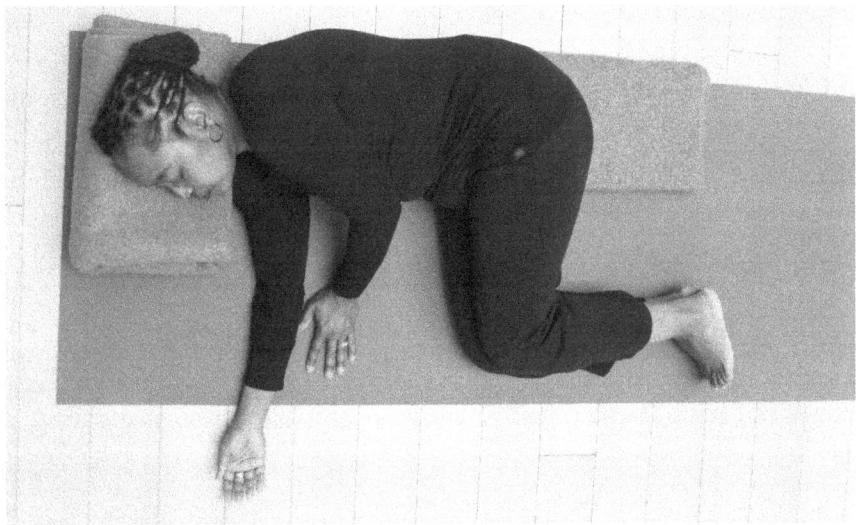

FIGURE 22: Side-lying savasana showing blanket support if needed due to discomfort of the bottom hip.

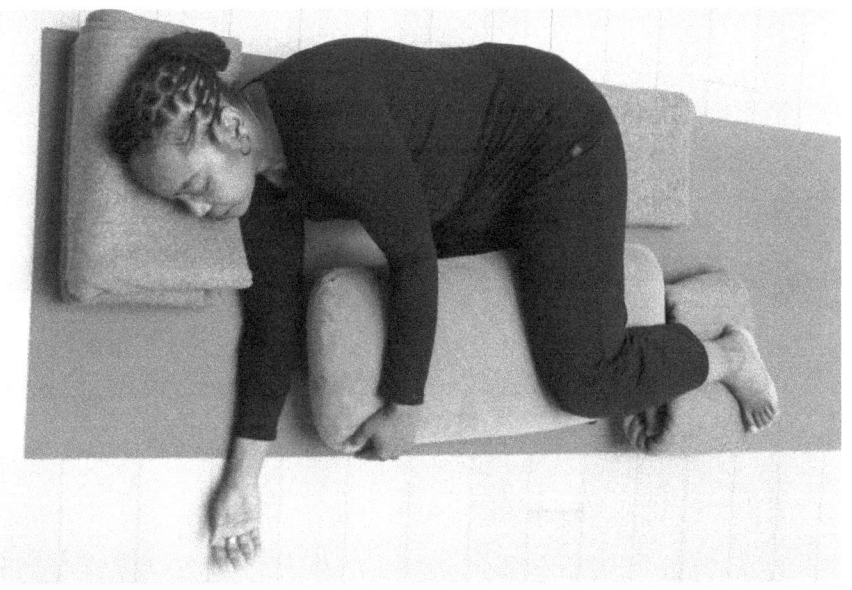

FIGURE 23: Side-lying savasana from above with all props.

3. Place the bottom arm straight out on the floor at shoulder height with the head resting on a folded blanket.
4. Slightly bend the knees and place a folded blanket or bolster between the thighs to reduce strain on the lower back and hips.
5. Ensure the neck remains neutral, avoiding tilting the head up or down.
6. Cover the eyes with an eye pillow or cloth and optionally cover the body with a blanket for warmth.
7. Rest the top arm in front of the torso or on a pillow, palm facing down.
8. Remain in this position for 10–20 minutes, allowing the breath to guide you into deep stillness.

Exiting the Pose

To come out of the pose, place your top hand on the floor and push yourself up to any seated position. Sit quietly for a few moments and observe.

Modifications

- If the bottom waist side feels collapsed, roll a small towel and place it under the side ribs for extra support.
- If the floor feels uncomfortable for your bottom hip, place a folded blanket under the hip.
- Resting on your right side can support relaxation by easing circulation and sometimes lowering blood pressure. When you rest on your left side, the position may encourage smoother digestion and help the body's lymphatic system flow more efficiently. Pregnant practitioners are encouraged to use the left side.

Seated Savasana in a Chair

Overview

There are times when reclining on the floor isn't feasible, such as when you have an injury or difficulty getting down and up. This seated savasana allows you to experience deep rest and stillness while supported in a chair setup. It can also be a useful variation for those with limited mobility or balance issues.

Props List

- Two sturdy chairs
- One yoga block (or a stack of hardcover books)
- One bolster (or firm cushion)
- One thick blanket

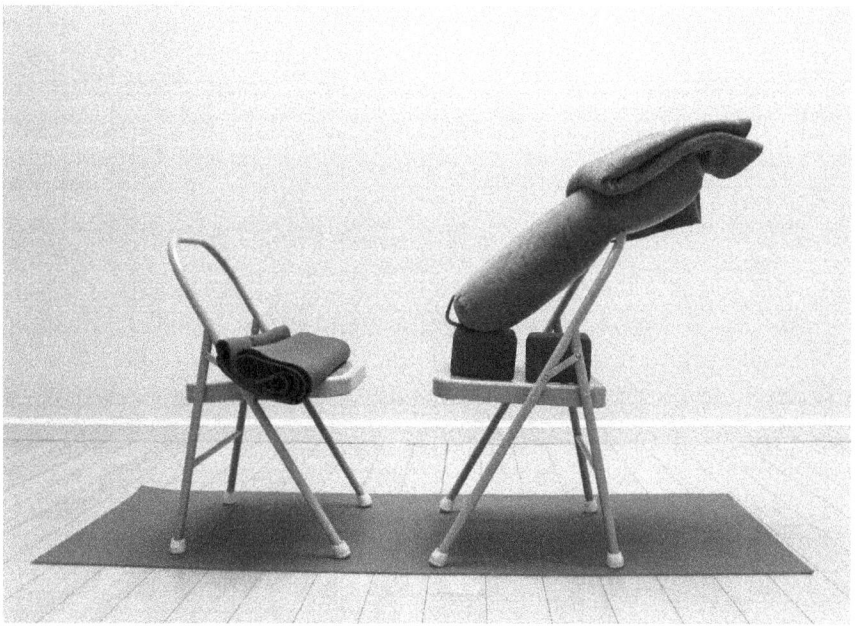

Prop setup for sitting savasana. Notice the padded seat on the chair to the left for the sitter. Notice on the chair to the right, a second block close to the back edge of the seat that will serve as a support for the arms

SAVASANA

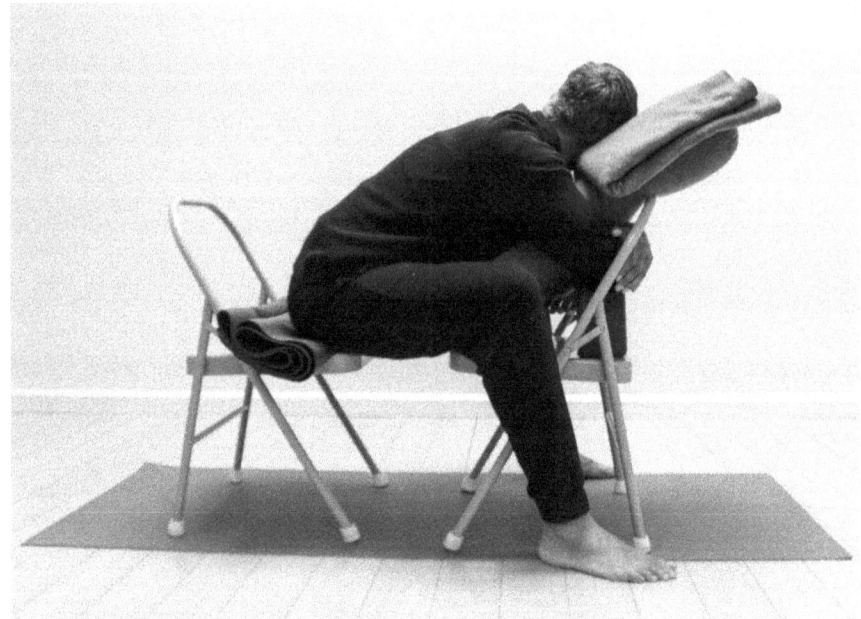

FIGURE 24: Savasana with chair. Notice how the second block is used to support the crossed forearms.

Instructions

1. Position the chairs: Place the two chairs facing each other with their front edges aligned. Adjust the distance between the chairs based on your height: taller practitioners may need more space, shorter practitioners may bring them closer together.

2. Sit on the front edge of chair 1, straddling chair 2 with your legs and feet.

3. Build the support on chair 2 by placing a yoga block (or stack of books) at the back edge of chair 2's seat.

4. Angle a bolster or firm cushion from the front edge of chair 2's seat across the top of the chair back to create a diagonal ramp supported by the block or books. If extra lift or comfort is needed, roll a thick blanket and place it on the bolster.

5. Fold forward and rest your torso on the ramped bolster. Slide your forearms beneath the bolster, cross them, and rest them on the block or book stack.

6. Turn your head to one side, resting it on the blanket-padded support. Try turning your head to both the right and left sides to find the most comfortable position. For regular practice, alternate sides each time.

7. Remain here for 5–8 minutes (or longer if comfortable), letting your breath flow naturally, as in traditional savasana.

8. To exit the pose, place your hands on your thighs and slowly bring your torso upright.

Using the Eye Wrap

The eye wrap can deepen relaxation in all versions of savasana by gently cueing the senses to turn inward. Note: Eye wraps are available online or at most Iyengar yoga studios.

Instructions

1. Begin with the wrap rolled up.
2. Hold the loose end lightly at one temple.
3. Unwind it slowly across the forehead, over the ears, and around the base of the skull.
4. Adjust the tension so it feels secure but not constrictive.
5. The wrap should provide a subtle sense of containment and quiet—not pressure. It softens light, quiets the senses, and invites the nervous system into stillness.

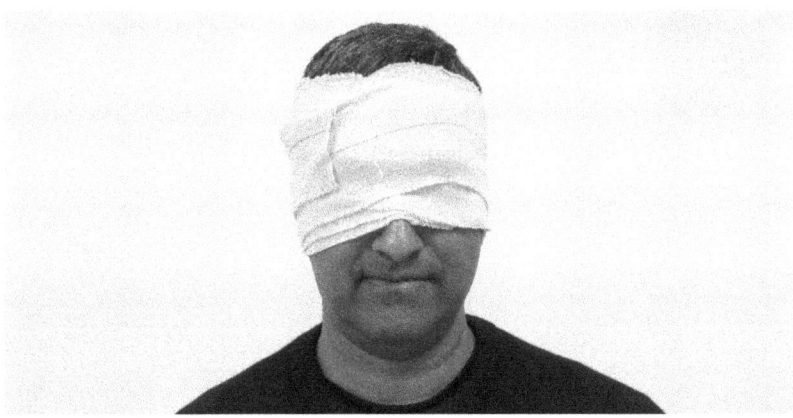

FIGURE 25: Eye wrap, which can be used in all versions of savasana. Notice the ears are also covered.

4 | How to Be in Savasana

The Paradox of Non-Doing

What's the difference between setting up the pose, getting into the pose, and being in the pose? The answer touches on one of the great mysteries of savasana.

Typically, asanas ask us to do something. This "doing" requires focus, strength, balance, and countless other elements. Savasana asks us not to do. It invites us to cease, to stop, to still. Even our language betrays the paradox: verbs like "stop" or "cease" still imply effort. But this is misleading.

Cultivating Conditions, Not Control

By properly setting up the pose—relaxing the body, calming the mind, and inviting subtle awareness, we create the conditions that might allow the pose's true potential to flower. We say might because it often takes time, patience, and grace before we arrive at that point. It's not something we do, it's something we allow to unfold.

At this stage, there are no specific instructions for being in the pose. Once the body is settled and the mind quiet, what remains is the witnessing presence that is already there beneath all activity. In yogic terms, this is consciousness. The closest we might get to guidance is "Stay present." Or perhaps, "Just be."

Our teacher Ramanand often guides us by repeating the phrase "I am," and ends with the final instruction: "Then let go of the 'I,' so that only the *'am-ness'* remains."

Why Savasana Often Comes Last

In the culinary world, some people espouse the idea of allowing certain foods to "rest" after coming out of the oven. As food cooks, moisture is pushed outward; resting allows the moisture to reabsorb. Flavors meld, the structure settles. The dish is more cohesive, balanced, and satisfying.

The same principle can apply to savasana at the end of a yoga practice. Regardless of whether it's vigorous power yoga, deeply supported restorative, or the precise alignment of Iyengar, savasana acts as that final, essential pause. It gives the body and mind time to absorb what just occurred. It's a practice of integration and reset before reentering the current of daily life.

After a sequence of postures that stretch, open, and energize, savasana invites us into stillness, allowing the nervous system to shift from sympathetic (fight or flight) to parasympathetic (rest and digest). In that quiet space, the work of the practice is metabolized physically, emotionally, and energetically. Thoughts, sensations, and feelings that surfaced during movement have room to settle.

In this quietude, the physical benefits of the practice are also more deeply absorbed. When savasana follows a yoga session, muscles, joints, and organs that have been stimulated and opened are given time to release residual tension, anchoring the structural and energetic shifts cultivated on the mat. As this tension releases and awareness moves inward, the deeper, more transformative qualities of savasana become available, and the inner landscape begins to reveal itself.

When Stillness Becomes Light: Leslie's Personal Experience

In over 30 years of practicing yoga, my most profound experiences have followed a well-crafted, deeply embodied hatha yoga practice. Several times over the years in my teacher Ramanand Patel's classes, something remarkable would happen. Why only in his classes is a mystery. It may have been something about his teaching, the depth of our relationship, or simply the immense love I carry for him as a longtime student. As I lay back into savasana, the space between my eyebrows (glabella) would begin to quiver. I would become unaware of this body-mind complex known as Leslie and would feel I was a ray of light, connected to everything in the cosmos. The next thing I'd hear was my teacher's voice, gently calling us back.

Those experiences became the inspiration for this book. I want everyone to have these moments in savasana. I had never felt such peace and connection. Even using the word "I" feels misleading—there was no "I." The vibration in the center of my forehead convinced me that the glabella, often referred to as the third eye that looks inward, or *ajna* in Sanskrit, is indeed real.

The Gift and the Mystery

When I had this savasana experience again, I asked Ramanand about it. He said it was a gift from the universe, and that I might one day see the "blue pearl."

Siddha yoga master Swami Muktananda described the blue pearl as "the light that illuminates the mind, that illuminates everything." Others have described it as containing the entire universe within the individual. I have not seen the blue pearl yet, but the classical yogic descriptions of *samadhi*, a state of complete absorption, come closest to describing what I experienced. In samadhi, one forgets the self entirely and merges with the infinite.

5 | The Still Point on the Path: Effort and Surrender

Savasana carries us beyond the physical, into the quiet center where practice becomes presence. It's where the mental, emotional, and energetic layers of practice come together. The pose shifts us from effort to stillness, from action to awareness. As the breath slows and the mind quiets, we may begin to witness thoughts, emotions, and sensations without identifying with them, a foundational tenet of yoga philosophy.

This witnessing presence, known in Sanskrit as *sakshin* or *drashta*, is our true nature: awareness itself. From this still place, the integration of our practice begins, and when we emerge, the peace and clarity cultivated on the mat can ripple into life beyond it.

More than 2,500 years ago, the Buddha likened the mind to a monkey, restlessly leaping from branch to branch. Fast forward to the digital age, and that monkey mind is now caffeinated and overscheduled. A widely circulated 2015 Microsoft report, popularized by *Time* magazine, claimed that our attention span has dropped to just 8 seconds, supposedly shorter than a goldfish's. Whether or not that number holds up scientifically, we can all sense its truth in how fragmented our attention has become. As teachers, we see this dispersion show up in our students' bodies, breath, nervous systems, and their ability to stay present.

Yoga and savasana offer a powerful remedy for that fragmentation, creating a moment when we can begin to weave the scattered pieces of ourselves back together. As British poet T. S. Eliot said:

> At the still point of the turning world. Neither flesh nor fleshless;
> Neither from nor towards; at the still point, there the dance is.

Eliot uses "the dance" to describe a stillness that transcends dualities, a dynamic pause at the center of life's movement. He captures the paradox at the heart of savasana: still, yet vibrantly alive.

Asana and savasana are part of a larger tapestry. The more we practice integrating that stillness, the more the lines between our time on the mat and our lives off the mat begin to be more permeable. That's where the practice becomes truly transformative.

Our teacher Ramanand Patel often said: "Leave the practice room quietly, and walk into the world with a savasana-mind." It was a reminder that the practice doesn't end when we roll up our mats. A savasana-mind lets us meet life with less reactivity and more ease, even if only for a few moments.

Some Savasana Is Better Than No Savasana

This, of course, begs the question: If we don't have time for a full asana cycle every day, can we or should we practice savasana as a stand-alone practice? And if we do so, is it substantially different? The most likely difference we will experience, however, is a result from what preceded the practice. If you've just completed a satisfying asana and breathing session, the body-mind, we might say, is primed for corpse. We've already released some degree of tension in our body, and our mind has been directed away from the cares and concerns of whatever's going on outside the practice room. When we practice savasana as a stand-alone pose at home, we usually don't have the benefit of such a yoga "warm up."

Equally important, as a beginner, it's fairly easy to slip into a corpse-like state when the wheels are greased by the expert guidance of a beloved teacher. Sometimes, even the sound of your teacher's voice can have a calming effect on your nervous system. Conversely, it tends to be more challenging if you're all by your lonesome.

Corpse pose is an "everyday" pose that should ideally be practiced, well, every day. Practicing it daily, even for just 10 minutes, will chip away at stress and rewire the nervous system into a more resilient, rested state. The benefits of savasana come not from intensity, but consistency.

The Indian sage Shri Aurobindo wrote: "All life is yoga." Whenever we choose to practice savasana whether it be at the end of a yoga practice, during a quick break from work, or at the end of the day—it will be part of the "yoga" of that day. Practiced regularly, savasana has the power to change your life.

The Paradox of Progress

The more experience we gain with movement-oriented asanas, the more we understand the subtlety and complexity of the postures. They become more challenging. Savasana progresses in the opposite direction. The more experienced we become at creating meditative space in us, the easier it will be for us to find our way into stillness.

Savasana is a stealthy pose. It unfolds quietly at first, asking you to trust that it's working. After a few weeks of daily practice, you may find that you are a little less reactive, a little more at ease.

Savasana calls for a quiet mastery: sustained focus, body awareness, a willingness to remain present without grasping or doing. These are elements cultivated slowly, through regular and intentional practice.

This integrative quality is what makes savasana so powerful. It doesn't just draw strength from other practices—it enhances them. Whether you are devoted to meditation, pranayama, tai chi, or any other body-mind practice, savasana acts as a bridge and a balm. All contemplative disciplines ultimately aim to foster calm, clarity, and presence. Savasana beautifully supports that aim.

6 | How to Exit Savasana
Because That's Just How I Roll

After stillness comes motion. The art of reentry and how we transition back to the world is as much a part of practice as the pose itself.

Here's a little story that is not true, but still worth pondering.

Once upon a time, a curious researcher hung a banana from the ceiling and placed a set of stairs underneath it. Then he let five monkeys enter the room. Before long, one monkey climbed the stairs toward the banana. As soon as he touched the stairs, however, the scientist sprayed all five monkeys with cold water. The monkeys learned their lesson quickly. The next time a monkey tried to get the banana, the others stopped him so they wouldn't get sprayed again.

The researcher then replaced one of the original monkeys with a new one. Naturally, the newcomer tried to climb the stairs, and the others pulled him down, even though he had never been sprayed. The new monkey learned not to approach the banana, though he didn't know why. Eventually, all the original monkeys were replaced, and none of the remaining monkeys had ever been sprayed. Still, every time a new monkey went for the banana, the rest would stop him. None of them knew why, they just did it.

Moral of the story? If we never question the "why" behind what we do, we risk becoming a case of monkey see, monkey do. Now, let's apply that to yoga.

If you ask a random yoga student—or even a teacher—why we

roll to the right when coming out of savasana, the response may be "That's just what I was taught." Cue the monkey story.

Some of the top U.S. yoga teachers offered compelling answers to my question about why we are taught to roll to the right. It's a surprisingly complex topic.

Why Roll to the Right? (or Not)

There's little historical context for the practice of rightward rolling, but yoga teacher extraordinaire Doug Keller offered this explanation:

> Of course, there are a lot of explanations that have to do with the positions of the heart and so forth. The one I always give, because it's most connected to tradition and makes the most sense to me, is when you roll to your right side after savasana, it keeps the left nostril open, the moon nadi, which tends to be more cooling to the body and helps you maintain a calm presence.... When the left nostril is more open, your blood pressure is a little lower, indicating a more parasympathetic state. Conversely, the right nostril (sun nadi) is associated with a more active, sympathetic state.

> Leslie: As a woman of a "certain age," I've found that during a hot flash, closing off the right nostril and breathing only through the left helps the heat dissipate quickly. Many of my students have confirmed that it works for them, too.

He goes on to say this nostril dominance is affected by the side you lie on, just like when you have a cold. Lying on your right side opens the left nostril. The shift in circulation is real.

Exit Stage Left?

Not everyone is on board with rolling to the right. Senior teacher and thoughtful rebel Judith Lasater said:

> When bringing folks out of savasana, I say, "Begin to notice the sounds and sensations in your body, the sounds around you. With an exhalation, bring your lower back ribs and the back rim of your

> pelvis down to the floor, turn your kneecaps to face the ceiling, drag one leg at a time up, put the feet on the bolster. Keep your lower back down, inhale, exhale, and roll to the side of your choice."

Wait, what? Roll to the side of your choice? I want the expert to tell me what to do! Judith has more:

> I've asked gynecologists, cardiologists, physiologists, and obstetricians why they want pregnant women to lie on the left; it's because the uterus can compress the descending aorta, reducing blood flow across the placenta. But for everyone else? I trust my students. They're coming out of a state of deep inner awareness. Listening to your body is part of the practice. Most people roll right, but I'm not sure how much of that is programming. I let them decide. I always feel an overwhelming urge to roll to the *left*. Rolling to the right never feels good to me, and that's how I deal with it.
>
> Trust yourself first. Notice I didn't say trust yourself only. But trust yourself first. Tune into your inner knowing. The teachings come through us, not from us. Our job is to listen to the cosmic grid and allow.

Other Teachers, Other Perspectives

Mary Paffard: "When I was in India, you rolled to the right for auspiciousness. But I don't think they really knew why. My right hip started getting irritated, so I began rolling to the left. It felt softer, less aggressive. More yin. I try to balance it out now."

Tias Little: "Sometimes I have students roll to both sides. Personally, I don't adhere to one side. Rolling to the right might help with blood flow through the liver or gallbladder, but it's so brief, the effect is minimal. When you stay longer on one side, it can affect the psoas and digestive organs. I think balancing both sides makes sense."

François Raoult: "No one really knows. Pregnant? Roll left. But otherwise? Right nostril, left nostril—it's all so subtle. Sometimes I think people feel what they're told to feel. It's called the subtle body for a reason—it's subtle. Putting a name on it can diminish the mystery."

So Which Way Do You Roll?

Clearly, there's no consensus. Maybe that's the point. If you have a heightened sensitivity and feel calmer when you roll to the right, great. If rolling to the left feels better, or is more accessible to your body, then that's your path. To borrow from Tias and Judith: Maybe it's best to balance it out and explore both sides. Trust yourself first.

The Inner Tools of Rest

The direction we roll may differ, but the destination is the same—inward. Yet for many of us, stillness doesn't come easily. When the body won't soften or the mind won't quiet, we can turn to three time-honored supports of breath, mantra, and mudra. Each offering a pathway to deepen stillness and sustain presence.

While savasana may be one of the crown jewels of the yogic path, it is not the only gem. Yoga offers many other practices with their own gifts—and their true power emerges in how they interrelate. You don't have to go deep into every one to feel their synergy. A little goes a long way.

PART II
Supportive Practices for the Restless and the Dying

7 | The Breath: Pathway to Stillness

Savasana is often described as the art of doing nothing. But anyone who has ever tried to lie down and just *be* knows it's not always that simple. Sometimes the nervous system is too charged to relax; sometimes the body can't lie down at all. For the dying, the ill, or those with limited mobility, the traditional shape of savasana may be out of reach, yet the essence of the practice remains available. The art of surrendering into stillness belongs to everyone.

If the nervous system is too revved up to relax, or the mind won't stop spinning, or the breath feels shallow and uneven, then achieving stillness may simply be uncomfortable. And for those whose bodies are weakened by illness or preparing to let go, stillness may take a different form entirely. That's where supportive tools like mantra, breath awareness, and mudra come in. These practices are not a distraction from the quiet of savasana. These practices will help lead us to that quiet.

For a restless mind, a mantra can be a gentle tether. When the breath is long and slow, awareness of its rhythm can begin to calm the nervous system. When energy feels stuck or unbalanced, a mudra can offer a subtle shift. Mantras, breath, and mudras. These are as-needed tools that are not intended to make us *do more*, but to help us *do less with more ease.*

Vayu Pratyahara: Drawing Inward

Vayu pratyahara is an ancient hatha yoga breathing technique. *Vayu* comes from the root *va*, meaning "to blow," and is often translated as air or breath.

Pratyahara, the fifth limb of the eight-limbed (ashtanga) practice outlined in the *Yoga Sutra*, is traditionally translated as "withdrawal," specifically the turning of the senses inward. It forms the bridge between the so-called outer limbs (bahiranga)—ethical restraints (yama), observances (niyama), posture (asana), and conscious breathing (pranayama)—and the inner limbs (antaranga) of concentration (dharana), meditation (dhyana), and absorption (samadhi). By drawing the senses away from external stimulation, pratyahara prepares the practitioner for deeper inward states.

Physically preparing for pratyahara calls for the following to essentially eliminate the distractions of physical movement:

- Assume a still but not rigid sitting position (asana, the third limb)
- Slow the breath way down (pranayama is limb four)

A helpful visual is that of a tortoise drawing its limbs and head into its shell. Through pratyahara, we prepare ourselves for the three so-called inner limbs of a yoga practice, a gradual intensification of meditation with the goal of self-realization.

The Breath: Drawing in the Wind

Drawing in the wind invites us to breathe, or imagine breathing, into parts of the body other than the lungs. Physically impossible, yes, but over time, the exercise sharpens our internal awareness in unexpected ways. Like many early texts, this one offers bold promises, stating that the practice can "destroy all diseases" and lead to full mastery of yoga. We advise taking that promise with a grain or two of salt!

But drawing in the wind is still a useful exercise for many reasons:

- It helps us consciously contact areas of our body that may not show up on our regular radar, strengthening our self-awareness.
- It asks us to use our breath in unusual ways so we gain a better understanding of ourselves as breathers. This can help us avoid falling into a "breathing rut."
- It helps us harness and soothe our scattered breath when we are in savasana. It calms our mind when we're ruffled by the proverbial "slings and arrows," a.k.a. stresses and strains, of "outrageous fortune," that is, the world.

The practice begins at your big toes and proceeds slowly upward through 18 stations known as *marmas* ("mortal spots") to end at the crown, or top, of your head. In the interest of making drawing in the wind a little more accessible, we've abridged it to nine stations, and made some substitutions. You can certainly add more stations once you've gained a level of comfort with nine-station drawing in the wind.

Nine Starter Stations

The stations we suggest you begin with are: Big toes → ankles → knees → perineum → navel → sternum → throat → glabella (between the eyebrows at the bridge of the nose) → crown.

You can experiment with how to breathe as you make your way through the stations. Here is one way to approach it:

1. At the first station, take a five- or six-count inhale.
2. Pause the breath there comfortably for a few counts.
3. Exhale for five or six counts.
4. Move on to the next station.
5. Repeat steps 1–4.

If stations are paired (big toes), be sure to breathe into both simultaneously. Don't overextend the pause at the end of the inhale. If your exhale "bursts out," then shorten the pause at the end of the inhale. Find a count that lets you release the breath softly and smoothly.

What happens if you reach the crown and those slings and arrows are still flying? Reverse the sequence and revisit each station back down to 1. Feel free to ascend/descend the stations as many times as needed.

Expanding the Practice: Seven Additional Stations

If you are ready to extend this practice and add stations, these next seven are optional.

- Mid-shin
- Mid-thigh
- Tail bone (coccyx)
- Mid-body, or *deha madhya*, the lower belly midway between the pubis and the navel
- Hollow or "well" of the throat, or *kantha-kupp*
- Root or base of the tongue
- Mid-forehead

You might also add a few stations of your own. Hardliners may howl at the idea of personal modification, but even traditions evolve!

There is one more station you might add, though it lies outside the body. In yogic tradition it is called the *dvadasha anta*, "the end of the twelve," and it's located about twelve finger-widths, or roughly a foot, above the crown of the head.

To explore it, direct your awareness upward from the crown into the space above you. Rest your attention there as if touching a subtle point of light or spaciousness. Some traditions regard this as a gateway, a threshold where the sense of self opens into something larger.

Spend a few breaths with this point if it resonates. Whether you imagine it as light, as space, or simply as an extension of your awareness, let it remind you that consciousness is not confined to the body.

Don't worry if some of these stations feel out of reach at first. If nine seems overwhelming, pare them down—even to just one. The Hindu sage Yajnavalkya, one of the early architects of yoga philosophy and a key teacher in the Upanishads, names three that can be practiced on their own:

- The sacrum that frees one from "bondage"
- The "internal space of the heart" that leads to the "highest state"
- The center of the eyebrows (glabella), where even a single breath held "for a second" unites you with the "highest state"

Yajnavalkya closes with an especially ambitious instruction: "Doing all your daily duties, focusing the prana in the center of the eyebrows, control it there till the mind is totally absorbed."

This is just one illustration of yoga's vast breath-based tool-set. The old yogis believed in adaptability, offering endless doorways to steady the mind, whether you are just beginning or far along the path.

8 | Mantra
The Sound That Carries Us Home

The Challenge of Repetitive Thought

Yajnavalkya's practice relies on imagination, which works well for some but not for all. Others may need something more concrete. This is where mantra comes in. A mantra is a sound or phrase repeated to anchor awareness, like a steady reminder that draws the mind back from distraction.

Unlike casual slogans ("You got this!"), a true mantra is intentional. From the root *man* ("to think") and *tra* ("instrument"), mantra means "an instrument of thought." In yogic practice, certain sounds and verses carry spiritual force, invoking clarity, courage, or devotion while quieting mental turbulence.

Repetitive thought loops often fuel anxiety and unease. Mantra helps break these loops, turning the mind's energy inward. As Patanjali describes, yoga is the stilling of the mind's fluctuations (*yogaś-citta-vṛtti-nirodhaḥ*).

Breath as Mantra:
Natural Sounds and Subtle Practice

How do we find a mantra for ourselves? Pause, close your eyes, and listen. Can you hear it? According to one yogic text, we unconsciously repeat a subtle breath-sound over 21,000 times per day—a natural, built-in mantra. From the moment we arrive in this world until we leave it, our breath carries this subtle sound.

To use the breath as a formal mantra, we amplify it slightly by constricting the throat muscles near the epiglottis. This achieves three things: it slows the breath; makes the sound more perceptible, to enable monitoring its quality (smooth or disturbed); and focuses awareness, reducing mental distractions. B.K.S. Iyengar notes the sound should resonate at the root of the nose and above the upper palate, and ideally remain even on both inhalation and exhalation.

Hamsa and *Soham*: Symbolism and Energetic Principles

How can the breath itself become a mantra, a "special sound" to anchor awareness? Yogis teach that each breath carries a subtle, natural sound: the exhale forms an aspirated *"ha,"* while the inhale produces a soft *"sa."* These imperceptible syllables reflect deeper truths about the Self.

Ha corresponds to *aham*, the Sanskrit word for "I," referring here to the spiritual Self (*jivatman*), the thread of conscious awareness. Symbolically, *ha* is linked to Shakti, the creative feminine force. *Sa* corresponds to Shiva, the witnessing masculine principle, or the universal Self (*paramatman*). Every breath, therefore, embodies the dynamic interplay of these forces.

These syllables can be joined as hamsa ("I am that") or soham ("I am that"), forming the ajapa mantra, the effortless, continuous mantra whispered by the breath. Soham is traditionally pronounced "so-hum," with a soft, resonant "m" sound that naturally aligns with the exhalation. The *Viveka Martanda* describes this mantra as a giver of liberation (*moksha*) for those who concentrate on it fully.

Om: The Primordial Sound and Its Spiritual Significance

As the breath deepens and quiets, the natural rhythm of hamsa may slow into a seamless pulse—*hamsa-aham, hamsa-aham*—eventually merging into the continuous vibration of om. In yoga tradition, *om* represents the unification of the individual self with the universal Self. Patanjali calls this vibration the *pranava*, the sacred utterance of Ishvara, the inner teacher or divine presence.

Om is also described as the "unstruck sound" (*anahata nada*), arising from silence itself, not from striking or rubbing objects together. All other sounds emerge from om, which contains all knowledge. When hamsa brings harmony to the breath, the combined mantras resolve into a continuous, waveless om, signifying the complete union of the individual and universal Self (Gorakhnath, 167; Patanjali, Yoga Sutra 1.27–29).

The Mandukya Upanishad describes *om* as:

> The past, the present, and the future, all that is simply *om*; and whatever else that is beyond the three times, that also is simply *om*, for that brahman is the Whole. Brahman is this self (atman).

9 | Mudras
Yoga in Your Hands

Introduction to Mudras and the Five Elements

In yoga, Ayurveda, and traditional Chinese medicine, the body is made up of five elements:

1. Earth
2. Air
3. Fire
4. Water
5. Space

Balance among them supports health, while imbalances may cause illness.

Nadis and Energy Pathways

- **Nadis:** Subtle energy channels carrying prana, the life force, throughout the body. Though there are over 40,000 nadis, simple techniques can help balance the elements and energy flow.
- **Mudras:** Hand gestures used worldwide in spiritual practices to influence energy. They can ease stress, support daily challenges, and help in end-of-life preparation.

Modern neuroscience now affirms what yogis have long intuited: The hands are portals to consciousness. A vast region of the brain

> **Accessible Adaptations for Illness, Aging, and Dying**
>
> For people with limited mobility, traditional yoga postures may be difficult or impossible. However, hand mudras are accessible to most individuals and can help reduce pain and improve breathing. Adaptations for stiff or arthritic hands, like using a washcloth or hair tie to maintain finger positions, can make mudras more achievable. Beyond physical benefits, mudras provide a point of meditation, which has been shown to ease pain.

is devoted to their movement and sensation, mirroring the ancient insight that prana flows where attention goes. When we form a mudra, we are literally shaping the mind.

Across traditions, sacred figures—from the Buddha's teaching gesture to Christ's raised hand in blessing—use the language of the hands to transmit meaning beyond words. Our palms have always been extensions of the heart, messengers of the soul.

Contemporary research echoes this wisdom: The hands occupy extraordinary neural real estate, with dense networks linking them to emotion, breath, and awareness. Research shows that the hands are deeply wired to our emotional and physiological well-being, making mudra a tangible bridge between science and spirit.

The Elements and the Chakras

In yoga, the shapes we create with our fingers in mudras guide energy through the nadis to the chakras, which are energy centers linked to the five elements of the body. The arrangement of fingers can increase, decrease, or balance a particular element: joining the fingertip with the thumb can amplify an element, while bending the finger toward the base of the thumb can reduce it.

The pelvic floor is the energetic center of the first chakra, *muladhara* (root), associated with earth. Earth governs muscles, bones, and stability. When balanced, we feel strong, grounded, and confident; when balance is lacking, we feel scattered or unsteady.

The sacrum and pelvic organs correspond to the second chakra, *svadhisthana* (sacral), associated with water. This element represents fluids, blood, and overall hydration. As we age, water diminishes, and imbalance may show as rigidity, emotional turbulence, or dryness.

The navel center is the third chakra, *manipura* ("city of jewels"), associated with fire. This is the seat of digestion, metabolism, and gut intelligence. When fire is strong, energy flows freely; when weak, one may experience digestive issues or feel mentally sluggish. Modern research supports this, showing how the "second brain" in the gut influences overall cognition.

The sternum is the fourth chakra, *anahata* ("unstruck sound"), linked to air (*vayu*). Air fuels respiration and circulation. Balanced air brings lightness, vitality, and emotional openness; imbalance can create tension or labored breathing.

The throat is the fifth chakra, *vishuddha* ("purity"), linked to space. Space is vital for air passage and expression. When balanced, we feel freedom and openness; when constricted, we feel restricted or blocked.

With this elemental framework in mind, it's not surprising that those who work closely with the dying often describe witnessing the elements "dissolve" one into another. The process begins as the earth element weakens, the body feels heavy and unsteady. As water leaves, the mouth and skin grow dry and the thirst intensifies. When the fire element wanes, warmth fades no matter how many blankets are added. As the air element departs, breathing becomes shallow and irregular until, at last, the last breath merges into infinite space. This ancient view of dying is not morbid but natural, reminding us that the same elements that animate the cosmos also compose and release us. Practicing mudra with elemental awareness prepares us to meet this transformation with awe rather than fear.

Experimenting with Mudras

Mudras can feel different depending on the pose, your state of mind, or even the day. They can be performed standing, seated, supine, prone, or even while walking; there's no single "best" way. With regular practice, mudras often deepen the breath and bring a subtle sense of ease to the body.

A few tips for practice:

- Pay close attention to the instructions, especially the subtle differences between connecting fingertips versus fingerprints. Precision matters—casual practice may reduce effectiveness.
- Hold only as much tension as needed to maintain the mudra. Fingers should come together naturally, not be forced.
- Although mudras can be performed in any position, symmetry helps. This could be savasana on the floor or bed, seated in a chair, or, if possible, in virasana (hero's pose).

How to Do Them

Before you practice, you may want to warm up your hands by clapping or by running warm water over them. The five fingers each represent an element and these five mudras correspond to the elemental body. See chart.

Prana and the Winds Within

In yoga, Prana is the life force that animates everything: breath, thoughts, digestion, and movement. Vayu means "wind" and refers to the many ways prana flows in the body. Two key movements are:

- **Prana Vayu:** drawing energy in and up (inhale, intake of food, ideas). Found in the chest and head. When it flows well, we feel alert and uplifted.
- **Apana Vayu:** releases energy down and out (exhale, elimination, letting go). Located in the pelvic floor and lower abdomen. Balancing apana supports digestion, detox, and emotional release.

Balanced prana and apana leave us energized yet relaxed.

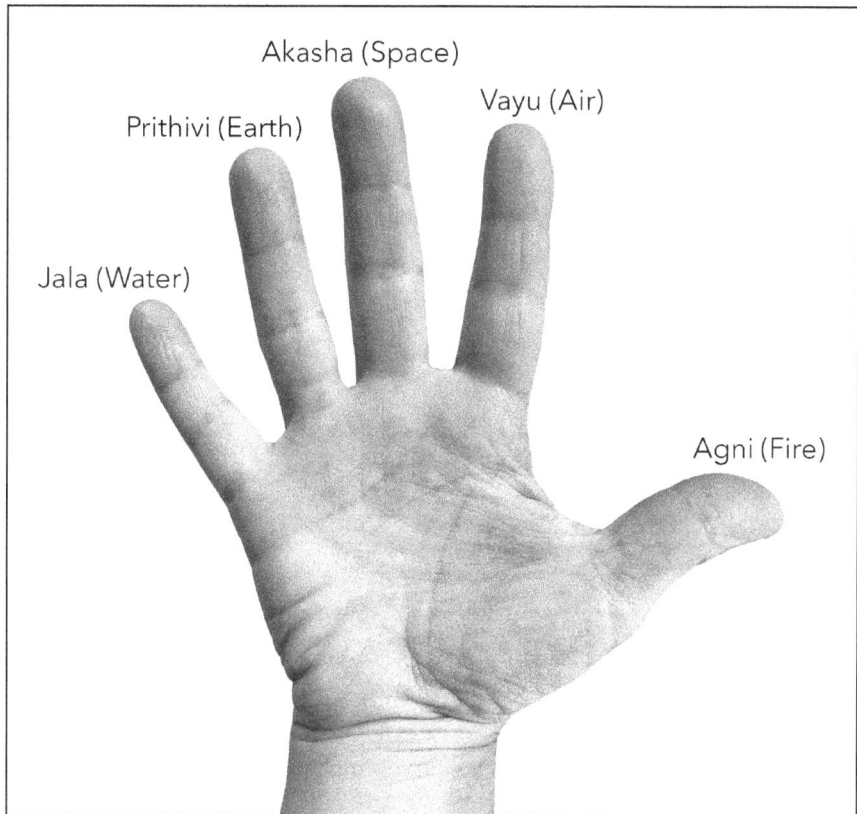

The elements represented in the hand.

Mudras to Support Prana and Apana

- **Prana Vayu Mudra:** Form a circle with thumb, ring, and pinky finger tips; index and middle fingers straight. Supports breathing, energy, calm, and clarity.
- **Apana Vayu Mudra:** Fold the index finger into the mound of the thumb, join thumb, middle, and ring fingertips; pinky straight. Supports digestion, elimination, and emotional release. Known as the "life-saving mudra."

Mudras help direct energy in the body, connect with the elements, and deepen awareness of breath and vitality.

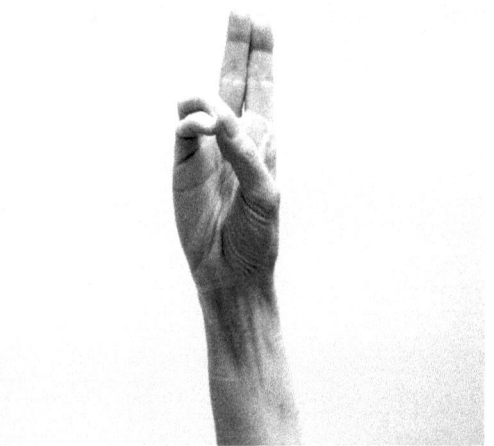 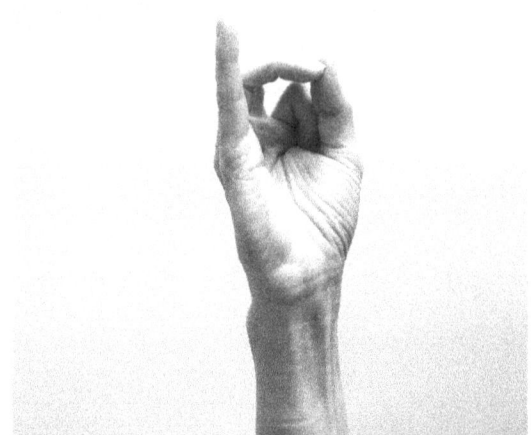

FIGURES 26A AND 26B: Prana Vayu Mudra (*left*) and Apana Vayu Mudra (*right*)

Prithvi Mudra (Earth Element—Muladhara Chakra)

- **Physical location:** The pelvic floor (perineum).
- **How to do it:** Touch the tip of the ring finger to the tip of the thumb on both hands. Keep the other fingers extended with minimal effort.
- **Benefits:** Balances the earth element and first chakra, grounding the body and mind. Supports stability, strength, and a sense of rootedness; especially helpful when feeling scattered or anxious.

Varuna Mudra (Water Element—Svadhisthana Chakra)

- **Physical location:** The area between the pubic bone and navel, front of the spine.
- **How to do it:** Touch the tip of the pinky finger to the tip of the thumb on both hands. Keep the other fingers extended and relaxed.
- **Benefits:** Balances the water element, supporting circulation, hydration, and emotional flow. Eases joint discomfort, dryness, or emotional imbalance, and nurtures creativity by harmonizing the second chakra.

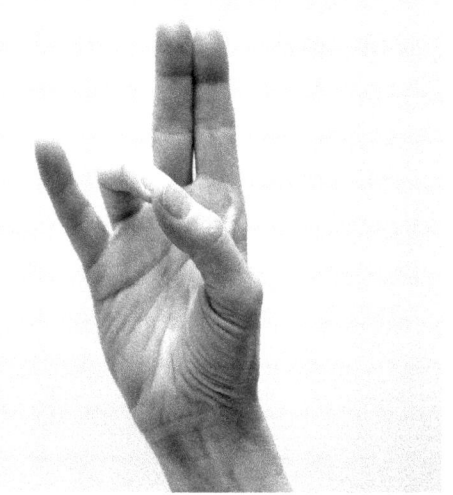
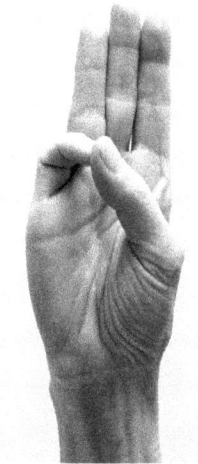

FIGURES 27A AND 27B: Prithivi Mudra (*left*) and Varuna Mudra (*right*)

Surya Mudra (Fire Element—Manipura Chakra)

- **Physical location:** The space behind the navel, in front of the spine.
- **How to do it:** Fold the ring finger to the base of the thumb and gently press it with the pad (not the tip) of the thumb. Keep the other fingers extended and relaxed.
- **Benefits:** *Surya* means "sun" in Sanskrit. This mudra activates the fire element, symbolizing the inner flame of transformation and liberation. It strengthens digestive fire, both physical and emotional, helping assimilate food or process challenges. In some traditions, fire is also associated with the heart center, representing the drive of a flaming heart toward enlightenment.

Vayu Mudra (Air Element—Anahata Chakra)

- **Physical location:** Behind the sternum, in front of the spine.
- **How to do it:** Fold the index finger to the base of the thumb, then gently press the side of the thumb against it. Keep the other fingers extended and relaxed.

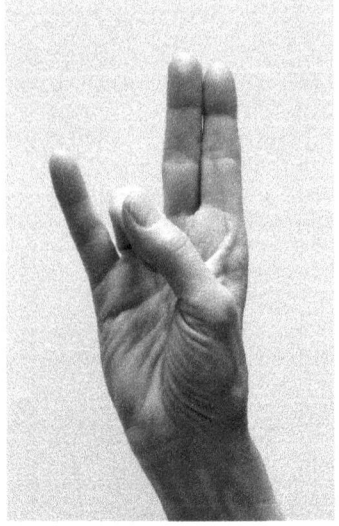 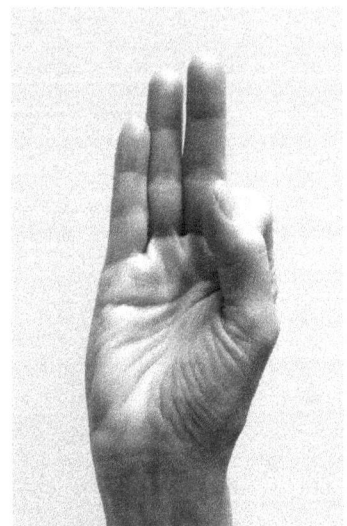 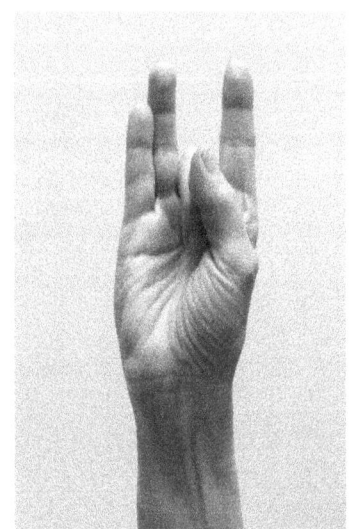

FIGURES 28A, 28B, AND 28C: Surya Mudra (*left*), Vayu Mudra (*center*), and Shunya Mudra (*right*)

- **Benefits:** *Vayu* means "wind," and the air element is associated with the heart chakra. This mudra supports the fourth chakra, promoting ease in the heart and lungs. It can help relieve anxiety, tension, grief, and respiratory discomfort, while gradually releasing chest tightness and deepening the breath.

Shunya Mudra (Space Element—Vishuddha Chakra)

- **Physical location:** Base of the throat, in front of the spine.
- **How to do it:** Fold the middle finger into the palm and gently press it with the thumb. Keep the other fingers extended and relaxed.
- **Benefits:** This mudra activates the throat chakra and the space element, enhancing openness, expression, and listening. It can relieve ear and sinus pressure and helps when feeling emotionally or communicatively constricted. Focus awareness behind the hollow of the throat.

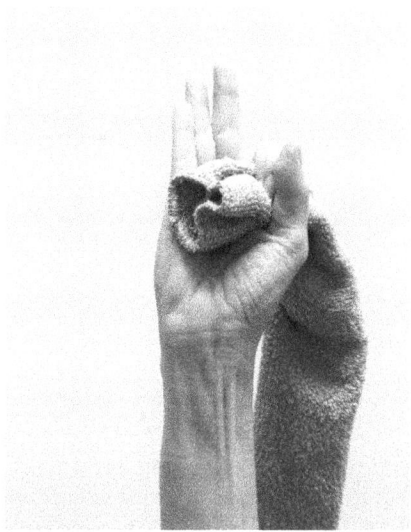 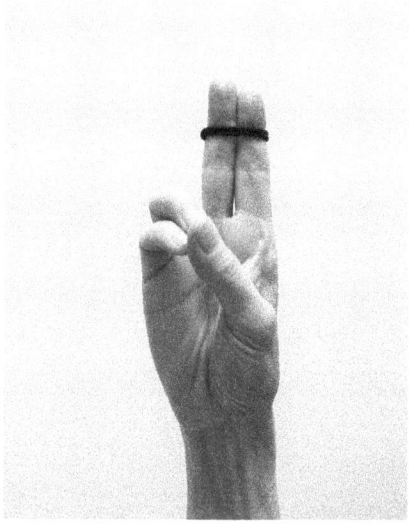

FIGURE 29: If you have difficulty with the shape of the fingers, try holding something soft like a washcloth.

FIGURE 30: If you have difficulty holding the fingers straight and together, try an elastic hair band.

Final Thoughts on Mudras

The effects of mudras are often subtle, more a whisper than a shout. Savasana, with its quieting of the nervous system, is an ideal posture for attuning to these finer layers of experience. Notice how your body and breath respond. Some mudras may feel more potent on certain days or in specific positions. Trust your sensations, and let curiosity guide you.

Tuning in to the subtle body cultivates a deeper awareness of impermanence. Everything is in flux, every breath, thought, and form.

This leads naturally to perhaps the most profound practice of all: Savasana, a pose that teaches us how to die so that we might fully live. More than rest, it is a gateway to presence, surrender, and letting go. In the final section of this book, we explore how savasana can help us meet the end of each practice, and the end of life itself, with greater ease, trust, and grace.

PART III
Death

10 | The Pose That Reveals the Path

> Yoga is to embody a limitless total presence. Ironically, to do this there must be a death. What dies is the singular, divisive, one-sided, erroneous self.... The death of the narrow mind itself is hard to come by, for no one oversees his own demise willingly—even if it is the death of that which causes us daily anguish and suffering. It is only when we are not looking and not in control that we can break through into "all-penetrating freedom" that "knows no blocks or barriers."... Thus we need the pose savasana to embody this profound letting go.
>
> — TIAS LITTLE, *The Practice Is the Path*

A well-worn proverb from one of Aesop's fables is "necessity is the mother of invention." We are more likely to do the work and figure out what needs to be done when we face a challenge. The "old yogis" certainly embody this proverb in what could be seen as the second greatest challenge after survival—our own mortality.

For the yogis of old, being born in a human body was a boon from the universe, a "precious wealth...no other form of body than human can pursue higher aims of life" (*Kularnava Tantra*, 1.18). For them, that was the purpose of life. Those yogis were in no hurry to leave this world created by the Hindu goddess Shakti, because life afforded a precious opportunity to realize our true selves.

Uncovering the secret of their mind-body's wealth was a matter of necessity. And everything the yogis needed to achieve that goal was right there if they (and we) could become still enough to access this wealth. Rather than fighting against and fleeing their own mortality, the yogis learned to accept it. Death was not the end.

Savasana as Threshold

> There is a third state in savasana that I call Ashunya. Shunya means "zero" in Sanskrit. The prefix A in A-shunya indicates a negation, so Ashunya means "fullness." Ashunya is what I call that state in savasana, and it is a state you only know when you are coming back from it. Students will occasionally say "I went somewhere."
>
> —JUDITH LASATER

Savasana, often mistaken for mere rest, can in fact be a portal to a liminal space that shares several key characteristics with another pathway: the transition from life to death. It is a profound practice for facing death and awakens the beauty of being human.

Through this lens, we'll explore Western and Eastern perspectives on mortality; ancient teachings on karma and reincarnation; contemporary Death Positivity movements; and how savasana can guide us into a more conscious, peaceful relationship with our own mortality. Our hope is to provide you with a full tool-set for understanding, preparing for, and embracing the power of the *last* savasana.

The work of dying is inseparable from the work of living. Through savasana, we touch the threshold between the two, discovering how intimacy with death can illuminate life itself. It can ease the fear and paralysis that often surround death by touching the primal source of love, kindness, and interconnectedness. "Zero" and "fullness," as Judith Lasater tells us, are etymologically very close to each other. We have all experienced the subtle space between being awake and falling asleep (science labels it *hypnagogia*). Throughout history, the most profound insights have emerged not from certainty, but from the spaces in between—neither here nor there, but rich with possibility. The yogic path invites us to be open to this deeper reality, not by transcending life, but by fully inhabiting it.

Death. An Open Question

> In savasana, we begin to train and educate ourselves for surrender.... Savasana simulates death and brings silence and non-movement. After all, what is death? It is a non-existing and a non-feeling state that one experiences often in savasana.
>
> —B.K.S. IYENGAR

What are some basic concepts of death per Western and Eastern traditions? Most Western perspectives agree on one point: Death marks the end of physical existence. Beyond that, however, there's little consensus. Is there something in us that lives on—a soul, a self, a consciousness, or some other essence that transcends death? And if so, in what form does it live on? In an afterlife, as in the Judeo-Christian tradition? As a return to a life force that will find other manifestations in ever new forms? If some aspect of us is everlasting, does it retain our individuality or dissolve into something larger?

Heaven Help Us Make Sense of It All

Our teacher Ramanand Patel, known for his clever humor, said: "Everyone wants to assure they will get to heaven, but no one wants to go."

In the Western tradition, two dominant views tend to shape the conversation about death. One is the atheist or existentialist perspective, which holds that death is the final end—no continuation, no afterlife, only nothingness. The other is rooted in the Christian worldview which affirms the existence of the soul, while Jewish tradition encompasses diverse views of what follows bodily death.

More recently, pantheistic and nature-based philosophies have gained renewed attention, emphasizing the deep interconnectedness of all things and the cyclical nature of existence. Here, death is not a termination but a return, a reabsorption into the great web of life, a merging with the source from which all things arise.

Time, in this view, is not linear but circular and rhythmic, echoing nature's cycles of birth, growth, decay, and renewal.

While this book cannot encompass the full sweep of Western thought on death, even a brief glance reveals how urgently and persistently the West has wrestled with mortality. The range and nuance of its inquiries, the sheer breadth of perspectives, underscores how central the question of our own end has always been.

Karma and the Long View of the Self

In the Eastern tradition, Hindu philosophy believes in an immaterial, eternal essence that survives the demise of our body. In the West, this essence could be the soul. In the Hindu tradition, the essence is the atman. Atman has three possible root verbs: "to move," "to blow," and "to breathe."

The Body: Blueprint of the Universe

In the yoga tradition, the physical body is a miniature version of the "body" of the universe. This implies that the universe itself has an essence, one that exceeds all human comprehension. It's omnipresent (everywhere), omnipotent (all-powerful), and omniscient (all-knowing). The Hindu tradition calls the universal essence, as it relates to the atman, paramatman, or the supreme atman. Each embodied atman is a fragment (amsha) of the paramatman.

The relationship between the atman and the paramatman is governed by karma, a word that has certainly become part of the modern cultural zeitgeist. What's important to know for our exploration is how karma is generated, how it affects the atman in the afterlife, and how it is overcome.

Karma has many definitions, but for us, it means "action." Action that covers what we do, what we say, and how we think. Our actions must have the proper intention; that is, they must be in line with a particular moral code and performed selflessly.

If we go into action with the intention of gaining something from it, however minimally and unconsciously, that action is ego-driven. We are attached to the action and the outcome. Seeing the world through ego-colored glasses distorts our perception of reality, prompting actions that are out of sync with the underlying order or "rightness" of the universe, also known as dharma. It's these "un-dharmic" actions that create karma.

Accumulated karma is not passive; it urges us to take more action of the same kind that created it in the first place. The newly acquired karma thus reinforces old karma and makes its urgency more compelling, and so we accumulate more karma. It's an endless loop: Karma creates more ego-driven action and the cycle continues.

You could think of karma as a cosmic credit card with no spending limit. Each ego-driven action adds to the balance. Even good karma racks up interest. Just like our credit debt, our karmic debt must be repaid. Sadly, most of us end our lives still in debt. In some versions of the afterlife, the atman stands before a deity in judgment. In others, no divine being is needed—karma itself serves as judge and jury and the verdict is always the same.

There is an old Elvis song called "Return to Sender." In other words, reincarnation or transmigration (punar janma), which roughly translates to "go back to existence." Once its karma is evaluated, the atman is provided with a new material body and sent back to the mundane world. Repeated reincarnations over countless lives is called samsara or "wandering through."

Why does karma still accrue if our actions are good? Good karma is certainly preferable to bad karma, but it's a debt. Even if we generate almost nothing but good karma, we're still returned to circulation. If the bad outweighs the good, our life might be a bit shorter and less happy. If the opposite, we can expect the reward of a fairly long and happy life.

Can I Jump off the Merry-Go-Round?

Is there some way "off" this karmic loop? Given that we all have free will, we have the possibility to pay off our karmic debt and free ourselves from samsara, that is, the self just jumping from one life to the next.

There are two key ways to exit the karmic carousel: *Behave appropriately.* Follow the rules for living with others and with yourself advanced by the various schools of yoga. These rules usually fall under two headings: *yama* and *niyama*. These are ethical guidelines, essentially, "dos and don'ts" to guide our behavior toward others (yama) and ourselves (niyama), as described by Patanjali in the *Yoga Sutra.*

Free ourselves from the misidentification with our ego. We're not talking here about doing away with the ego, just redefining our relationship with it so we no longer confuse it with what its Latin root implies: "I." Instead, we can dedicate, maybe even sacrifice, our actions to the "Absolute"—whomever or whatever we believe exists at the heart of the universe.

In other words, sacrifice of the self (small *s*) invites the guidance of the Self (capital *S*). This is what the Bhagavad Gita calls *naishkarmya karma,* or karma that transcends karma. When our deeds are free from ego-based grasping and dedicated to something greater than ourselves, they stop generating new karma. We can begin to resolve the karmic debt.

Now we must not assume that if someone's life is difficult, it is a consequence of all their bad karma. That shows a lack of compassion and a gross misunderstanding of karmic philosophy. None of us can see into another person's karmic history; we do not know what led to the individual being in their present situation. Perhaps the sacrifice we should make is that, if we meet someone whose life is in shambles, we help them out as best we can. That will serve our karma well.

11 | The Liminal Space
Coming Home

> Tinkerbell: "You know that place between sleep and awake, that place where you still remember dreaming? That's where I'll always love you, Peter Pan. That's where I'll be waiting."
>
> —J. M. BARRIE, *Peter Pan*

Savasana is a practice of transitions; a practice that allows us to linger in a space we otherwise experience primarily between waking and sleeping. The descent into sleep is *hypnagogia*. The ascent from sleep into waking is called *hypnopompia*.

These in-between states are fleeting yet rich with altered perception. As defined in both scientific and popular literature, these states are known to give rise to vivid imagery, fragments of lucid dreams, and even experiences of paralysis or a sense of presence. Fascinatingly, similar phenomena are often reported near the end of life: visions, sounds, and a dissolving of the usual boundaries between self and other. What the dying encounter and what we may occasionally glimpse in savasana may belong to the same mysterious terrain.

The liminal space briefly entered during such transitions has long been revered as a portal to deep insight and transformation. Visions are the most commonly described, but auditory and tactile experiences also occur. One of my yoga students once described hearing choral music in savasana—so vividly that he assumed a neighbor had turned on a stereo.

Others have described the sensation of being suspended in a timeless void, where there is no separation between self and environment, only stillness and spaciousness. I once sat with a hospice patient who could not understand why I wasn't hearing the beautiful music surrounding her. When I asked what she was hearing, she smiled and said it was the traditional Hebrew hymns she had sung as a child in synagogue. For her, this was not a hallucination. She had pierced a veil between worlds.

That is what the practice of savasana prepares us for, the thinning of the veil. It teaches us to become still enough to listen, open enough to receive, and spacious enough to allow something greater to move through us—whether it is silence, a vision, or an ethereal melody from our past.

There are countless stories of loved ones appearing in the days or hours before death—guiding, comforting, or simply being present. These visitations, often dismissed as dreams or delusions, may in fact be profound crossings of awareness. They echo what some practitioners encounter in savasana: a meeting with presence beyond time.

Eric Small, a senior Iyengar yoga teacher, recounted visions of his teacher, B.K.S. Iyengar, and lineage that arose for him while in the pose:

> I was always very conscious of his image in front of me. And I saw him in a very real sense. But I think my breakthrough was when I then saw Krishnamacharya [Mr. Iyengar's teacher] standing behind him. And then I saw another man standing behind Krishnamacharya. It was like seeing cards on a table, Mr. Iyengar and his teachers standing behind him.... It was very comforting. They were not so much watching over me as coming toward me, their influences and their essences.

When the body is allowed to relax, it can slip into this threshold state within moments. In Sanskrit, the word *sandhya* refers to *twilight*, a symbolic bridge between day and night, breath in and breath out—a metaphor for the transition between consciousness and unconsciousness.

This in-between realm, this liminal state, is a powerful place to linger. Roger Cole, PhD, a long-time Iyengar yoga instructor and expert in sleep medicine, likens this in-between state of savasana to "an ancient forest, it's been there for so long, holding still for so long that everything is coming into its own balance without anyone directing it. And so our own mind, if we just leave it alone, will come into its own equilibrium. A lot of the benefit of savasana is allowing it the time to take place."

Where Do We Go When We Are Asleep?

> I've had the experience of dropping into different states of consciousness, a certain awareness of the body as being absolutely motionless and at the same time feeling spacious and empty—as if I would go back and forth between not even being able to feel the body and then coming back and feeling it once again. And having that as an experience of a deeper state of consciousness. A sense of energy moving through what the yogis call the nadis. It felt like a cleansing and a holistic awareness of the body, but it was accompanied with deeper and deeper states of awareness in savasana that felt like I was on the margin of consciousness.
>
> —DOUG KELLER

There is a substantial body of research affirming how essential rest and sleep are. "Sleep plays a vital role in good health and well-being throughout your life. The way you feel while you are awake depends in part on what happens while you are sleeping. During sleep, your body is working to support healthy brain function and maintain your physical health," according to the National Institutes of Health website (NIH, "Why Is Sleep Important?," accessed Sept. 10, 2025). B.K.S. Iyengar wrote in *Light on Life* that "in deep sleep, we touch the divine."

Sleep is a return to the Self (capital S) that quietly persists beneath all fluctuations of thought and feeling. This is the essence of who we truly are—not our bodies, thoughts, emotions, or identities, but the unchanging awareness that perceives it all. This deeper Self is the awareness that observes your breath, absorbs these words, and remains constant through every shift in emotion or experience yet is not tied to what comes and goes, it simply exists. It dwells for a time in the temporary home of the body and continues beyond the body when we leave it.

In an effort to give students a sense of this awareness, our teacher Ramanand Patel asks us to think of that delicate threshold we cross as we return from the depths of sleep to waking life. In that fleeting moment, we awaken not as ourselves, but simply as awareness. We do not remember our name, our story, or where we are. It is a rare instance of pure consciousness, untouched by the weight of self.

This moment offers a subtle and sacred glimpse of the threshold we may cross at the time of death. Just as in that liminal state between sleep and waking, the constructed self begins to dissolve. What remains is the witness—still, spacious, and aware. Practicing this kind of presence in savasana prepares us to meet death not with fear, but with familiarity.

The yogic path is not about escaping life but about awakening to this deeper reality while fully inhabiting our bodies and our lives. We are less rattled by the highs and lows because we remember where home truly is. Ramanand says the true meaning of savasana is a going home. This is not an intellectual idea. It is something we feel, something we become aware of in the practice itself. And it is in this recognition, in this anchoring in the truth of who we are, that real liberation begins. Not freedom *from* life, but freedom *in* life.

12 | Practice Dying and Do It in Savasana

Mathematically, I think it's zero. You are in a state of zero needs, zero desire, close to zero mental and physical activity. A quiet zero state of awareness without perspective.

—RODNEY YEE

Whether we look forward to an upcoming event or whether we dread it, the quality of our experience is influenced by how we prepare for it and by how well we are prepared. Particularly when we anticipate that an event may be painful or challenging, it helps to become familiar with how it might unfold. We can imagine it in advance, anticipate possible difficulties, and allow space for greater ease and steadiness.

The exercise below is intended to help you become more comfortable with your own mortality. Its core approach can be adapted across a variety of practices—for example, during meditation, or when reflecting quietly on your own journal keeping. More immediately, it's set up to be practiced during a yoga asana and breathing practice, but you can adjust it to any practice you follow.

Lie down in a savasana-like position.

- Close your eyes and feel the touch points of your body against the ground that supports you.
- Sense the back of your skull resting on the earth.
- Notice your upper back, arms, and hands where they meet the floor.
- Feel how your pelvis and buttocks rest.

- If your knees are supported, acknowledge the sensation of the backs of your knees resting.
- Finally, sense the back edges of your heels touching the ground.

As if watching yourself in a film, begin to visualize your body resting on the earth, fully supported. Acknowledge that while you have a body, you are not the body itself.

Now, turn your attention to your breath. Take a few moments to observe the length of each inhale and exhale. Do not attempt to manipulate your breathing, allow it to follow its natural rhythm. With each inhalation, notice any areas of the body that feel restricted or tight. Gently invite those areas to release their tension.

Once your breath is calm and your body relaxed, imagine yourself in a doctor's office. You haven't been feeling quite like yourself lately, and after running some tests, your doctor shares the results: Your time is limited, and you most likely have only a few months to live.

What thoughts arise upon hearing this news? What sensations ripple through your body? What emotions surface—fear, sadness, anger, perhaps relief or curiosity? Or maybe a sense of numbness? There is no right or wrong reaction; simply stay with whatever emerges, without judgment.

You leave the doctor's office and sit in your car, letting the news sink in. Do you feel the urge to call someone? If so, who? Are there people you would not want to tell? And if so, is it because you want to protect them, or because you do not want to care for them in this moment?

Now fast forward a few months. Everyone in your life knows about your prognosis. It is becoming harder to care for yourself, and your world feels smaller as going out is no longer easy. Who do you want around you at this time? As your health and strength decline, do you feel more afraid of dying, or less?

Finally, imagine your death is imminent. You are lying in bed, unable to move or speak, but still aware of your surroundings. Who is with you in these last moments? Picture the scene. Are you at home? You hear yourself being cared for; your physical needs are met. Turn inward now: Are you ready to let go, no longer able to communicate outwardly? Do you sense peace, acceptance, curiosity, or perhaps fear and resistance? Again, there is no right or wrong answer.

After sitting with this reflection, bring your attention back to the breath. Feel the support of the floor or chair beneath you. Allow the sounds around you to drift effortlessly into your awareness; let hearing happen on its own. When you open your eyes, let seeing arise naturally, without effort.

When you are ready, gently leave the pose and take time to journal about your experience. If you find it difficult to remember the sequence, record the guidance on your phone for playback, or ask a trusted friend to read it to you slowly.

Repeating this process can take you deeper into your thoughts and feelings. It may bring clarity about what is left undone or unsaid—matters you still have time to address. It is also a practice in letting go. With repetition, you may find a growing sense of ease, perhaps even joy.

13 | Let the Reaper out of the Closet

If you want to unsettle your dinner guests, suggest talking about death. The silence that follows or the awkward change of subject says everything. Death is rarely considered suitable for polite conversation; talking about your own death is, well, let's just call it a showstopper.

The avoidance is understandable. In our culture, death conjures exactly what we are taught to resist: fear, loss, futility, painful memories. What good could possibly come from talking about that? At best it feels pointless, at worst morbid. Even for those who pride themselves on being rational and unsuperstitious, death-talk carries an unease—as if giving it words might somehow invite it closer.

This refusal, however, becomes most problematic when death is no longer abstract. Sitting at the bedside of someone who is dying, many of us search for anything—small talk, medical updates, even denial itself—rather than name what is happening. In hospitals, doctors may emphasize treatment plans over honest conversations about quality of life. Death, rather than being acknowledged as natural, is framed as a medical failure.

Woody Allen once quipped: "I'm not afraid of dying, I just don't want to be there when it happens." The same could be said of conversations about dying; we want the subject kept at arm's length. But this avoidance creates a profound dissonance. We pretend, even in the very presence of death, that it is not here.

I think we need to be clear that our unwillingness to be open and real about death is outright harmful. It creates tremendous suffering because it cuts off many vital opportunities to alleviate our fears, share and support one another, benefit and learn from others' experiences.

It also stunts our personal growth and chokes the flow of compassion and understanding. Our lives could be richer and more meaningful if we embraced the reality of our mortality.

This truth is not new. Followers of Stoic philosophy taught that freedom comes from meditating on death, not to obsess over non-existence but to live more vividly. Seneca urged us to rehearse death daily, so that we might treasure the ordinary hours we are given. Yogic philosophy echoes this. Patanjali names ignorance (*avidya*), attachment, and clinging to bodily life as root causes of suffering. To see clearly, including our own finitude, is the path to freedom.

So how do we begin to see clearly? How do we allow death into the conversation, not as an intruder but as a companion? How do we grow curious about it, learn from it, even allow it to soften and transform us?

Encouragingly, a cultural shift is already underway. Since the 1970s, hospice and palliative care have helped countless people die with dignity. The Death Positivity movement invites mortality into daily life, while Death Cafés gather strangers around tables to speak of dying as openly as living. Death doulas now offer guidance and companionship at the end of life. Step by step, the conversation is changing.

For me, death entered quietly through the doorway of my yoga practice. Over time, savasana stopped being just "the final pose." I began to recognize it instead as a teacher of presence, a rehearsal of letting go, a mirror of impermanence woven through every breath. Death was no longer distant or dramatic—it was already here, informing life from within.

The poem "Color of the Sky," by Tony Hoagland captures this shift:

What I thought was an end turned out to be a middle.
What I thought was a brick wall turned out to be a tunnel.
What I thought was an injustice
turned out to be a color of the sky.

So much of what we fear as finality is simply unfamiliar territory. Everything is transition. Life is not fixed; it is fluid, sky-like, ever-changing. When we remember this, we soften. We stop clutching. And in that release, we begin to really live.

Memento Mori on the Mat

> In deep relaxation... savasana, we may have an experience of the infinite small or the infinite large—a sense of space, lightness, and luminosity.
>
> —FRANÇOIS RAOULT, *My Lifeasana*

The guiding principle of my yoga practice is to deepen awareness. Awareness in yoga isn't confined to the physical. It includes an intimate recognition of our thoughts, emotions, breath, and how we move through space. Awareness is limitless. To exclude death is to misunderstand the very aim of the practice: to quiet the mind, see clearly, and awaken to the truth of who we are.

Savasana reminds us that someday we will die. It is a practice run for the real thing, a place to glimpse dissolution, expansion, or oneness.

Asked about his experience with the infinite small and infinite large in savasana, Raoult explained:

> Yes, well, if you lose yourself and have to touch your skin to make sure you're still there, it's similar to what they talk about in physics—you get an experiential glimpse of it. We are more space than anything else. The space part of you connects with the space that is everywhere.

This isn't just a spiritual metaphor; it's a scientific fact. We are made of atoms, each one a cathedral of space. An article from

Interesting Engineering posits that if the nucleus were the size of a peanut, the atom itself would stretch the length of a baseball stadium. That's how much of us is emptiness. Our bodies, though they feel solid, are mostly just space.

That same spaciousness, the vastness between nucleus and electrons, lives in the subtle spaces of our lives. It is the pause between each breath, the stillness before the next thought arises. In savasana, we slip into these small openings and discover not absence but expansion. When we stop striving, narrating, becoming, we open into being. And being, as it turns out, is vast.

Paradoxically, it's in the briefest, most fleeting thresholds that we encounter the eternal. Just as physical atoms are mostly space, so too are our days held together by small, invisible intervals, tiny deaths, subtle endings, moments of non-doing.

Impermanence gives these spaces their depth. Without the limits of time, we would not recognize spaciousness at all. Even the most magnificent sunset would become tedious if it never ended. Its beauty lies in its brevity. Temporality heightens our awareness. Through the fleeting, we glimpse the infinite.

While we all understand this, most of us don't live with it in the forefront of our minds. Rather, we endlessly look at our phones (thanks to infinite scroll) and act as if we had all the time in the world. Endless availability kills preciousness.

Imagine approaching a yoga pose with the awareness that it might be your last time ever feeling it. You'd want to drink it in fully, to experience its vibrancy, texture, and aliveness. Even if we're not quite that dramatic, we can still arrive in the pose with the intention to fully inhabit the present moment. This simple act of attention breathes life into the practice. Awareness of temporality is what lets a moment shimmer. Without impermanence, nothing is sacred, because everything is assumed to always be there.

The more we can be in the moment, the more we experience a felt sense of no-separation. This is the overarching goal of practicing yoga. The more we become aware of the changing nature of everything, the more deeply we connect with that which is immutable.

To cultivate this awareness, we don't need to meditate over a corpse or volunteer in hospice, although those can be noble acts. Daily life and yoga practice offer ample opportunities. There are many ways to die, and death is only one of them. We shed identities, release attachments, let go of illusions—all of which prepare us for the letting go that awaits us all.

In facing the temporal, we touch the eternal. In staying present, we rehearse the deepest letting go. But until that moment, we can support one another with compassion, presence, and a shared awe for the mystery of being alive.

We are also part of a larger collective facing this same mystery. While the yoga mat offers us an intimate space to explore death inwardly through the breath, the body, and the quiet magnitude of savasana, how we live and how we die is shaped not just by personal practice, but by culture. In recent years, a shift has begun. Just as modern yogis are reclaiming death as a sacred teacher, a new cultural movement is emerging, one that invites us to meet mortality with honesty, creativity, and even community.

14 | The Death Positivity Movement

> For what is it to die but to stand naked in the wind and to melt into the sun? And when the earth shall claim your limbs, then shall you truly dance.
>
> —KAHLIL GIBRAN, *On Death*

Yoga is a practice of cultivating awareness that invites us to see more clearly and respond with greater care. In savasana, that awareness extends to dying itself: a rehearsal in letting go and in seeing clearly the impact of our actions, even beyond our own lifetime. The Death Positivity movement invites us to carry this consciousness off the mat—into how we relate to death personally, culturally, and ecologically. In the yogic tradition, this reflects the principle of *ahimsa*, non-violence. Ahimsa is the commitment to live and die in ways that cause the least harm. Caring for the earth, even in our final acts, becomes a continuation of our practice.

The term "death positivity" is attributed to Caitlin Doughty, a Los Angeles–based funeral director who saw how the funeral business, some have called it the "funeral industrial complex," took advantage of the vulnerabilities of those "left behind" after a loved one's death.

Doughty made it her mission to educate people and offer new options around burial via an organization she called The Order of the Good Death (hereafter known as the Order).

It wasn't too long ago in the United States that most people died at home. Family members tended to the body, wrapped it in a cloth, and transported the coffin to the cemetery. The 19th century heralded the handover of death from families to what became the funeral industry, thanks to societal changes such as urbanization and laws governing various aspects of burial, according to the blog "Evolution of American Funerary Customs and Laws," from the Library of Congress (accessed Sept. 17, 2025).

According to Doughty, the Order is about making death a part of your life. That means committing to staring down your death fears, whether it be your own death, the death of those you love, the pain of dying, the afterlife (or lack thereof), grief, corpses, bodily decomposition, or all of the above—accepting that death itself is natural, but the death anxiety and terror of modern culture are not.

The Order became a hub of "death-centric" artists, including fashion designers who make compostable garb for the recently departed, eco-makeup artists, and body composters. The movement hopes to "be the change" it has introduced.

In fact, a noticeable shift is happening around all things death—societally as well as individually. It's beginning to dawn on us just how much we can benefit from doing death differently.

The Death Positivity movement is the next evolution of Doughty's brilliant vision.

Death Doulas: Ushers to the Nearest Exit

An end-of-life or death doula is "a nonmedical companion who provides personalized and compassionate support to individuals, families, and their circles of care as they encounter and navigate death, loss, and mortality. An end-of-life doula advocates self-determination and imparts psychosocial, emotional, spiritual, and practical care to empower dignity throughout the dying process," according to the International End of Life Doula Association.

My yoga teaching and practice have been suffused with the understanding that *we are not the body*, that *we are simply passing through*, and that has made me receptive to the idea of the work of a death doula. Guiding others as they prepare to leave this temporary dwelling felt like a natural extension of my teaching. Not long after hearing about it, I signed up for a death doula training.

Little did I know the extent to which this training would open my eyes to the wealth of possibilities tied to dying: preparing for it, getting comfortable with it, helping friends and family with the loss. When we take the time to educate ourselves, explore our options, and speak openly, death becomes less a crisis and more a rite of passage.

I invite you to take a number at the "Death Deli Counter." You may find you'll be better prepared when your number is called.

Death Café

My death doula instructor mentioned the term "Death Café." Various surreal images immediately popped up for me: Day of the Dead (Día de Los Muertos) skeletons and grim reapers swapping stories over espresso and biscotti.

Of course, that's a scene from a Halloween display. There is no physical place called a Death Café, although it is a shared space, physical or virtual, where people come together to talk about death, sometimes over coffee and cake. The Death Café is an invitation to "increase awareness of death to help people make the most of their (finite) lives," according to the Death Café website (accessed Sept. 17, 2025).

The concept can be traced back to the "café mortel" movement, started by Swiss sociologist Bernard Crettaz. British electrical engineer Jon Underwood, a self-described "death entrepreneur," hosted the first official Death Café in his London home in 2011. Since then, these gatherings have spread worldwide (Underwood died in 2017 at age 44 of an undiagnosed blood cancer, according to an obituary in *The Guardian*).

To be clear, Death Cafés are not grief-management groups. They're not therapy sessions. Rather, they are informal, participant-led conversations that range from the philosophical to the practical: What does a good death mean to you? Should we compost bodies? Are headstones outdated? No agenda. No selling. Just open-hearted, death-curious dialogue.

And they are often full of laughter. I started a monthly Death

Café at an Oakland yoga studio called Nest Yoga, and after 2 years, what continues to strike me is how much levity, relief, and camaraderie emerge. People tell stories, crack jokes, share fears. There's cake, and sometimes there are tears. There is always honesty.

At nearly every gathering, there are variations on the same theme:

- "This is one of the only places I can have a truly authentic conversation [about death]."
- "It's such a relief to talk about death without people squirming."
- "I saw how my partner struggled at the end. I don't want to die like that."

One woman introduced herself and then announced she had terminal cancer. Instead of automatically offering sympathy and well wishes, we all just listened to what she shared. When she finished, she said: "I just want to thank you for NOT saying 'I'm sorry.'" She was tired of being pitied. What she craved was connection without platitude, companionship without denial.

These are the kinds of conversations we rarely get to have in everyday life, and yet they're essential.

Authenticity. Self-awareness. *Svadhyaya* (self-study). One-pointed attention. Conscious dying. These are the great questions of yoga philosophy. Death Cafés offer us a modern way to practice these ancient inquiries—one slice of cake, and one brave conversation, at a time.

Conscious Dying

Death and dying can be painful, at times agonizing, and it's natural to want to ease that suffering. In modern medicine, this is often achieved through heavy sedation, especially in the final days of life. This approach definitely offers relief, although at a spiritual cost of the loss of awareness in the final moments. For those who value clarity and presence, this raises powerful questions: Can

Just Put Me in the Green Bin

Ahimsa, meaning non-violence or non-harming, is one of the most important yogic principles and the ground from which all others grow. Non-violence is the recognition that we are all interconnected: What we do to others or to the planet, we do to ourselves. After we shed the body like a worn garment, what to do with it?

Parallel with death positivity is the idea of opting for more environmentally sound after-death "homes" for the body. Some of these more planet-friendly options are:

- **Human composting:** Composting with wood chips and straw. The body will decompose in about 30 days under wood chips and straw.

- **Eco-friendly caskets:** Made of biodegradable and sustainably sourced materials such as bamboo, willow, seagrass, pine, cotton, cardboard, and wool. No toxic finishes, such as glues or varnishes, are used.

- **Eco-urn:** A container for cremated remains made from natural materials that will decompose naturally in soil or water over time.

- **Reef burial:** Cremated remains are mixed with eco-friendly concrete and molded into a reef-like structure that is placed on the seabed, creating a new marine habitat.

- **Burial suit:** A biodegradable garment, most likely embedded with mushroom mycelium and spores that act as decomposers.

- **Tree burial pod:** Cremated ashes are placed in a biodegradable urn or pod and planted with a tree.

These are just a few options from a list that will no doubt expand over time, although your choices may vary depending on what part of the country or world you reside in.

dying be more than something we endure? Can it be something we do, consciously?

Centuries-old global spiritual traditions have urged us to consider the importance and sacredness of this moment of transition. In Tibetan Buddhism, the dying are asked to do three things at the moment of death:

- Release all grasping and aversions
- Keep the heart and mind pure
- Unite the mind with the mind of the Buddha

Some examples of on-the-verge-of-death rituals include receiving deathbed teachings via a monk reading sacred texts during and after death (Buddhism); offering final confession and receiving last rites from a priest (Catholicism); receiving holy water from the Ganges or having a priest read from holy texts (Hinduism); and reciting a confession prayer followed by the *Shema*, the affirmation of God's unity (Judaism). Regardless of the method, the intent is similar: to go out with a pure heart and a clear conscience.

Even for those who hold no religious or metaphysical beliefs, there's still reason to value awareness at life's end. This final moment belongs to you. Why surrender it to fear or sedation when it could be met with curiosity, clarity, and a deep, wordless presence? According to the Bhagavad Gita:

> Worn-out garments are shed by the body: worn-out bodies are shed by the dweller within.... New bodies are donned by the dweller, like garments.

Yoga teaches that our true Self is not the body but the eternal witness within. When the outer layers fall away in the moments of our transition, maybe our spiritual Self becomes unencumbered, freed from the constraints we carried with us, pure. Why would we not open ourselves to that possibility? What have we got to lose?

Ultimately, how each of us meets death—whether through the relief of medication, with the aid of medical assistance, or through conscious presence—is deeply personal. There is no single right way to die, just as there is no single way to live. What matters is that our choices reflect our own values, comfort, and understanding. Whether we seek rebirth, heaven, or simply peace, conscious dying invites us to align our final breath with our deepest truth.

Epilogue

> In B.K.S. Iyengar's *Light on Yoga,* savasana is the only pose that has no number of difficulty. It is difficult to face yourself in a silent state. You are confronted with a void. When you are totally still, you have a witness inside of you. You are nonexistent.
>
> —FRANÇOIS RAOULT

What begins as stillness on the floor may become one of the most courageous acts of all: to stop, to feel, to witness. What began as our simple inquiry into savasana, a pose many see as just lying still, has given rise to a profound meditation on living and dying. Savasana may just be the most auspicious pose of all.

In its classical form, savasana was considered a practice of dissolution, a mini rehearsal of the final exhale, a homecoming of sorts. The *Hatha Yoga Pradipika* describes it in the simplest possible terms:

> *uttanam savavabhumau sayanam tacchavasanam*
>   lying on the ground like a corpse, that is savasana

No embellishments. No grand philosophical explanations. Just lie down and stop moving.

The practice of savasana reveals the interconnectedness of our heart, our mind, and our physical body. The practice of stillness helps us become aware of our breath and the life force that it carries. It can show us the pain we hold and guard in our body. When we sense the pain, we breathe into it; doing so is sometimes enough to release it.

With regular practice, savasana helps us witness our thoughts, our emotions, and our sensations at the same time reminding us that we are *not* our thoughts, emotions, and sensations. Through practice and grace, savasana can show us that we are both the observer and the observed. It offers a vantage point where there is nothing left to fix, no role to play, only being.

In this state of deep stillness, where the layers fall away—body, mind, story—a question may quietly arise, not as a thought, but as a felt inquiry.

Who Am I?

Koham is Sanskrit for "Who am I?" Esteemed sages have said that it is the *only* question truly worth asking.

This is not a philosophical trick question. It's a question born in the silence of savasana. When we're no longer doing, becoming, performing, what remains? Who is the one aware?

Consider the experience of watching or participating in a play, where actors fully embrace their characters. At times, we can become so absorbed in the performance that we momentarily forget it's just a play. In life, too, we become identified with our parts: I am a teacher. I am a spouse. I am this body. Yoga philosophy teaches that we are far more than the roles we assume. Experiencing this realization can transform how we see ourselves and the world around us. This new perspective allows us to view life—and death—in a way we never have before.

There is an answer to the question, "Who am I?" It's *soham*, or "I am that."

> *tejo yat te rūpaṃ kalyāṇatamaṃ tat te paśyāmi yo 'sāv asau puruṣaḥ so'ham asmi*
>> The light which is thy fairest form, I see it. I am what this is.

—UPANISHADS

Our Invitation

Take a deep breath. Let go. Become the witness to all of it.

When the time comes for your last savasana, may you meet it not with fear, but with ease, knowing you've been practicing all along.

And for the love of all that's sacred...

Don't leave class early.

APPENDIX
Teaching Savasana:
For Teachers and the Just Plain Curious

As a beginning teacher, there are two things you ideally do before teaching savasana to a class.

1. **Convince yourself that savasana is essential.** We assume that you've already come to this conclusion since you've purchased this book and have read some, most, or all of it. But if you're on the fence, we hope this book has helped you decide in favor of the pose.

2. **Convince your students of its value.** Savasana can be a difficult sell. Students may resist because of the off-putting name, which for Westerners can make them uncomfortable or because they see it as "doing nothing" and a waste of time. Ironically, those who most need savasana are often the students who have pushed themselves hardest in class.

For new classes with beginners, it's easier: These students have no entrenched bias against the pose. Early on, prepare a short remark to answer the common question: Why am I doing this? Acknowledge the pose's unusual nature and explain its purpose and benefits.

In established classes, you may encounter resistance if your predecessor wasn't savasana-friendly. Never criticize another teacher; maintain professional respect.

Key Reminders for Every Practice

- Savasana is a true asana and should be treated with the same care and attention as any other pose.
- Even minor movements, like scratching an itch, disrupt the stillness of the brain.

Deliver your instructions clearly and briskly, especially if the time for savasana is short, ensuring students spend as much time in silence as possible. Bring them out of the pose with extreme slowness to avoid abrupt transitions back to the external world. Some teachers even recommend maintaining silence until leaving the practice room.

Always leave time for savasana, even if it means shortening the active practice. Encourage students to practice savasana at home regularly, individually or with partners, friends, or family. But participation should never be forced. Savasana is the gift at the end of the practice; it's the big bow on the yoga package.

Adjusting Your Students

Always ask permission to touch someone, even if they told you last week it was okay. With all hands-on work, always begin by asking for permission, especially with new students. A simple, *"Do you mind if I make a small adjustment to your shoulders?"* is enough. Wait for a clear "yes" before proceeding.

Shoulder Blade Adjustment

This adjustment almost always brings a smile of relief to the face of the student receiving it. While this adjustment can be done from the side of the student's body, it is most effective facing the student head-on. This requires straddling their torso, so be mindful that not every student will feel comfortable with this positioning. If needed, adapt your stance to maintain professionalism and safety.

To Adjust:

- Position your feet on either side of the student's waist and lean forward. It doesn't matter which shoulder you begin with, but it's often best to start with the non-dominant side. Since most people are right-handed, begin with the **left shoulder.**
- Slide your **right hand,*** palm up, between the student's side torso and inner arm until it rests under the shoulder blade.
- At the same time, place your **left hand** on the head of the upper arm bone (humerus).
- Spread your right palm gently and begin to draw the shoulder blade downward.
- Simultaneously, gently press the humerus head toward the floor with your left hand.
- As you slide your right hand out from under the shoulder blade, use your left hand to guide the student's arm into a gentle lateral (outward) rotation.

Repeat the same sequence on the **right shoulder**, reversing your hands. You may need to apply slightly more pressure on this side, but remain cautious. **Firm yet gentle** is the key.

Once both shoulders are adjusted, they should appear more even and relaxed away from the ears. To finish, you may return to each humerus head for one final, grounding press, light, steady, and reassuring.

Base of the Skull Adjustment

Once the shoulders are in place, you may notice that the student's head is slightly tilted or askew, perhaps the chin lifts subtly toward the ceiling due to tightness at the base of the skull.

---

* As you're facing them, your left and right will be opposite to theirs.

To Adjust:

- Kneel behind the student's head and slide your hands underneath to cradle the back of the skull in your palms.
- Carefully lift the head just an inch or two off the floor.
- Use your fingertips to find the lower edge of the occiput, where the skull meets the nape of the neck.
- Gently press into this border and apply a slight traction, drawing the occiput away from the neck.
- Hold this traction for 10–15 seconds.

When finished, slowly and mindfully lower the head back to the floor, making sure it doesn't thump down abruptly.

Leg Adjustment

Creating a sense of length in the legs and hips can offer immediate relief, especially in the lower back, sacroiliac region, and hip joints. This adjustment helps the student feel both grounded and spacious.

As always, work with minimal effort in your own body. For this adjustment, sit a few inches away from their feet in *upavistha konasana* (seated with legs wide). When leaning back, maintain a neutral spine to protect your own back.

To Adjust:

- Position yourself at the foot of the student's mat.
- Slide your hands beneath the student's ankles so that your fingers cradle the Achilles tendons and your palms wrap lightly around the heels.
- Gently lift both legs off the ground—just an inch or two, no more than necessary.
- As you lift, apply light but steady traction, drawing the legs away from the hips. Imagine the movement as a long, gentle exhale.

- Pause briefly at the peak of the stretch, letting the student's body register the sensation of length and release.
- Slowly lower the legs back to the mat with the same smooth, intentional movement, ensuring the return feels as supportive as the lift.

Words Matter

Keep in mind that your language in savasana can impact the student experience.

Possessive Language

Example: "Relax your hand."

- **Advantages:**
  - Creates personal ownership and easier connection with the body
  - Feels nurturing and direct
  - Helps new or less body-aware students identify and release tension
- **Disadvantages:**
  - Can reinforce attachment to the body, counter to surrender
  - May reduce the sense of universality
  - Could trigger resistance in trauma-sensitive settings
  - May feel too intimate for some students

Neutral Language

Example: "Relax the hand."

- **Advantages:**
  - Encourages detachment and observation
  - Supports a meditative, universal experience
  - Helps students who focus too much on pain

- **Disadvantages:**
  - May feel impersonal or less engaging
  - Can be confusing for beginners or those with low body awareness
  - Might not resonate in warm, personal teaching environments

Setting-Specific Language

- General yoga classes: Possessive language may offer more accessibility
- Meditative/advanced settings: Neutral language may encourage surrender
- Trauma-sensitive classes: Neutral language preferred, but some gentle possessive cues may help
- Balanced approach: Read the room. Alternate between possessive and neutral language

Cueing Styles

Declarative Cueing

Example: "Relax your forehead."

- **Advantages:**
  - Clear, direct guidance
  - Effective for beginners
  - Efficient for quick transitions
  - Empowers students to actively relax
- **Disadvantages:**
  - Can feel forceful
  - May encourage effort rather than natural release
  - Less suited for deep meditative surrender

Invitational Cueing

Example: "Allow the forehead to relax."

- **Advantages:**
  - Encourages surrender and aligns with savasana's essence
  - Gentle, reduces resistance
  - Supports nervous system regulation
  - Trauma-sensitive
- **Disadvantages:**
  - Less direct, may confuse beginners
  - Can feel vague
  - Works more gradually, not ideal in short classes

Setting-Specific Cueing

- Beginning/structured classes: Declarative for clarity
- Meditative/restorative/trauma-sensitive: Invitational for ease
- Both: Start declarative to create awareness, then shift to invitational for deeper surrender

Sample Savasana Scripts

If you normally don't say anything when your students are in savasana, you can use these scripts until you find your own words. We don't have a set script and always vary what we say. Depending on how much time you have, make sure you pause between instructions. The ratio of talking to quiet should be about 50/50. Lead them in and then let them be. We feel it is important to balance guidance into savasana and silence for simply being.

Script 1

It's time for savasana.

If you'd like, place a bolster under your knees. This encourages the heads of the thigh bones to settle into the hip sockets, which in turn softens the groins. When the groins harden, the natural rise and fall of the torso with the breath can feel restricted.

If your chin is lifting toward the ceiling and you sense compression at the back of your neck, place a folded blanket under your head. Ideally, the underside of the chin should rest more or less perpendicular to the floor. This releases the base of the skull away from the neck and allows the throat and tongue to soften.

Let your tongue settle on the floor of your mouth. Widen it gently from its midline, letting the sides drift down and back into the throat. Tias Little calls this "tongue savasana."

Place your feet hip-width apart and let them turn outward evenly from the hips. With your hands, lightly "scrub" or slide the back of the pelvis downward through the tailbone. This helps free the lumbar spine, without flattening its natural curve.

Broaden the shoulder blades and draw them down the back, toward the tailbone. Balance that by widening the collarbones across the chest. If you like, use your fingertips to press gently beneath the clavicles—lifting them slightly from the upper ribs before softening them outward. *Clavicle*, from the Latin *clavis*, means "key"; these are the keys that open the eyes of the heart.

Allow the upper arms, the humerus bones, to sink into the shoulder joints, just as the thigh bones nestle into the hips. Sense the four corners of your torso—both shoulders and both hips—anchoring into the earth.

Lay your arms out about 45 degrees from the torso. Too high and the shoulders may lift; too low and the ribs cannot expand freely. Turn the palms to face upward and let the fingers unfurl.

Ensure your head is neutral. The ears equidistant from each shoulder, the eyes balanced in relation to the floor. Let your body rest without touching anything unnecessary.

Now imagine the eyes sinking into the back of their sockets. Smooth the skin of the face, especially the forehead, allowing it to broaden outward toward the temples. In your mind's eye, imagine the brain shrinking and settling at the back of the skull. Shrink, sink, and release. No thinking required—thinking stiffens the brain.

Let the whole body yield to gravity. Feel your back as if it were warm oil poured into a skillet—spreading, settling, sinking.

If you feel the urge to fidget or scratch, do it now. Later, try to remain still. If you must move, keep it minimal and then return to square one.

Stay with yourself. Notice the breath. If the mind wanders, gently guide it back without judgment. The breath is your anchor.

If settling feels difficult, begin with 8 to 10 slow, steady inhalations and exhalations. Then return to a natural rhythm. Let the breath breathe itself. Notice if you're holding anywhere—gripping the throat, tightening the belly. If so, soften. No need to fix or force anything, just notice and rest.

This is savasana.

Script 2

Let's allow the body to rest now, let everything you've just done in your practice metabolize.

If you need support under the head, place a folded blanket beneath it. Everyone should take support under the knees, even just a rolled blanket or bolster; it helps release the lower back and groins. If you think you'll get cold, cover yourself with a blanket. If you have an eye cover, use it. It can help you drop into relaxation more easily.

[Pause briefly to allow students to adjust]

Now, take a moment to check your alignment. Savasana is a real pose—alignment matters, even here.

Begin with the pelvis. Notice if one side of the buttocks feels higher towards the head than the other. If so, lift the pelvis slightly and use your hands to draw the flesh of the buttocks down and away from the lower back. This lengthens the lumbar spine and helps create symmetry.

Bring your attention to the shoulder blades. Can you feel them evenly grounded on the floor? Is one shoulder bearing more weight? If so, gently roll that shoulder under until your chest feels broad and open.

When you feel that the body is as symmetrical as possible, bring your awareness to the breath.

Can you feel the animation of the body as you breathe?

With each inhalation, sense the body widening, spreading outward from the center to make space. With each exhalation, feel everything softening back toward your midline.

Now feel or imagine the crown of the head and the tailbone moving slightly away from each other with each inhale, releasing toward each other on the exhale.

Picture the central channel of the body, your primary energetic line, running just in front of the spine. Place your mind there. Envision a column of light or energy, subtle but radiant, aligned from the base of the tailbone to the crown of the head.

With each inhalation, imagine this light extending just beyond the physical body, above the head and below the tail.

With each exhale, feel it drawing gently back inward, consolidating into that central line.

If there's any part along that central axis that feels blocked, heavy, or unclear, invite a sense of clarity there. Imagine unobstructed energy, pure light, flowing freely up and down your spine.

Feel the whole body resting into the earth. Feel the weight of your feet, your legs. The softness of the belly. The openness of the chest. The weight of the arms and hands. The gentle stillness of the face.

Let yourself fully rest. Let go. Just be.

Bringing Students out of Savasana

To come out of savasana, bring your attention to the feeling of your body resting on the ground. Before moving, imagine you are above yourself, just witnessing. Observe this image of yourself on the ground, breath animating the flesh, noticing the thoughts that float through.

Then, bend your knees one at a time and roll onto your side. Pause there. Curl in slightly and rest for a few breaths.

When you're ready, press yourself up slowly using whichever

hand is on top, allowing your head to lift last. Sit quietly for a moment with your eyes closed and bring to mind something in your life for which you are grateful.

May the calm of savasana stay with you as you move into your day (or evening).

BOOK CLUB QUESTIONS

Part I—The Pose

1. How did your understanding of savasana change after reading this section?
2. The authors describe savasana as both "a pose and a path." What does that mean to you?
3. Have you ever experienced a moment in savasana that felt deeper than simple rest? What conditions helped create it?
4. How might you integrate savasana as a stand-alone daily practice, rather than only as an ending to asana?

Part II—Supportive Practices for the Restless and the Dying

5. What does "effortless effort" mean in your own yoga or meditation practice?
6. How do breath, mantra, and mudra serve as tools to settle the nervous system or support you in moments of transition?
7. Which supportive prop or variation of savasana resonated most with you, and why?
8. How might these practices be adapted for someone who is ill, dying, or caring for someone at the end of life?

9. How does the idea of the "witness" (sakshi) help you relate to thoughts or emotions that arise during stillness?
10. In what ways do the teachings on prana, the elements, and the chakras shape your view of what it means to be alive—and to let go?

Part III—Death

11. How does savasana serve as a metaphor for death and for living consciously?
12. The book invites readers to explore mortality without fear. How do you personally feel when contemplating your own death?
13. How does the principle of ahimsa (non-violence) inform your choices about the earth, the body, and the way we approach death?
14. What aspects of the Death Positivity movement align with yogic philosophy, and where might they diverge?

Closing Reflections

15. What practices or insights from this book do you feel most drawn to integrate into your life?
16. How has this exploration of savasana changed your understanding of yoga as a whole?
17. What does "not leaving class early" mean to you—both in yoga and in life?

ACKNOWLEDGMENTS

Turns out, doing nothing well takes a whole team. Looking back at my notes, I've been working on this project since 2007—so it's a long road of thank yous on this journey.

I bow in deep gratitude to the many teachers, friends, editors, readers, and colleagues who helped bring this offering to life.

Uber-mega thanks to Jürgen Möller, who once again worked his organizational magic to herd my sprawling notes and untamed ideas into a coherent narrative. This would not, could not have happened without you.

To Hannah Moss, master of the visual pose, this book would not breathe as clearly without your photographic eye. To Kim Lally and Nest Yoga, for always being supportive, generous, and affirming.

My gratitude to the teachers who generously shared their time and insights for this project: Rodney Yee, Genny Kapula, Judith Lasater, Tias Little, Doug Keller, François Raoult, Roger Cole, Eric Small, Mary Paffard, Patricia Sullivan, and Annie Carpenter. Your voices added richness and depth.

To Richard Rosen, whose wit, wisdom, and long game with the breath have been a steady compass throughout this project. This book is all the richer for your gift with words, your deep scholarship, and your wry humor.

A heartfelt nod to my editors—Shalmali Pal, Lucy Smith, and Bill Anelli—for wielding red pens with love and rigor, and not letting me off the hook when clarity was hiding.

Big *namaste* to my thoughtful early readers: Carla Koop, Cynthia Doubleday, Susan McCormick, and Anne Blackman for catching the rough edges and polishing the message.

To Sabrina Chaumette and Arun Rao, your grounded presence in our photos inspires us to drop in more fully. And to Katarzyna Kopańska, whose exquisite, ethereal art graces our cover, thank you for capturing the spirit of this work.

To the death-aware and savasana-curious communities, the hospice teams, the Death Cafés, and the students who've shared, "That savasana was profound"—thank you for affirming that stillness is not an absence but a portal.

To Erin Oliver and Kaiser Oakland Hospice for the opportunity to guide folks to the door. And to all my hospice patients who have allowed me the honor of being with them until the end (of this life).

To my guiding yoga light, Ramanand Patel, gratitude as vast as the sky for showing me the way. I love you with my heart.

And finally, to the teachers before the teachers. To the unseen lineage that quietly holds the space between breath and death, thank you for whispering, *"Lie down. Let go. Listen."*

INDEX

Acceptance— as gateway to peace, 77, 81–86; as surrender, 77

Ajna (third eye)— awakened experience of, 51–53; energetic center of insight, 70

Alignment—physical and energetic, *various savasanas*; teacher reminders, 1132–15

Anahata (heart chakra)—Part II, Ch. 7

Apana Vayu—downward-moving life force, 72, 73–74

Asana—meaning of, xiv, 3–8; savasana as, 9–11

Awareness—cultivation of, 66–68; as witness consciousness, 81–90

Ayurveda—five elements and balance, 69

Bardo—liminal state between life and death, x, 87–90

Body— as microcosm of universe, 81–87; as vehicle for consciousness, *various savasanas*

Bolsters—uses for support, 10–11, *various savasanas*

Breath—bridge between life and death, 61–66; as mantra, 66–68

Buddha—postures of stillness, ix

Chair savasana—setup and adaptations, 32–35

Chakras—relation to elements and mudras, 70–71

Clarity—arising from stillness, 53, 66

Corpse pose— as rehearsal for dying, 81–86; symbolism of, xiv, 4–6, 9–11, 52–53

Death—as transition not end, 81–107

Death Café—community dialogue on mortality, 95, 101–2

Death Positivity movement—modern reframing of dying, 95, 99–105

Dream states—relation to savasana, 87–90

Effort and surrender—paradox of, 10, 48, 51–53

Elements—relationship to mudras and chakras, 69–77

Energy pathways (nadis)—69–70

Equanimity—in savasana and death practice, 87–90

Exiting Savasana—options and traditions, 54–57

Eye wrap—use for quieting the senses, 47

Faith—arising when reason dissolves, x
Forehead weight variation—to quiet the mind, 28–31
Freedom—as release from self, 87–90

Glabella—focus between brows, 30–32, 50
Grace—meeting effort, 51–53; surrender into, 91–93
Grounding— breath as grounding, 61–65; through props and weight, 12–47
Guru lineage—honoring teachers, 88, 126

Hatha Yoga Pradipika—earliest text on savasana, 4
Head support—proper setup for alignment, 13
Heart—opening through breath and awareness, 75–76; rolling to the right, 42, 55

Impermanence—reflection on, 77, 95–98
Inner stillness—cultivating, 9–11, 49, 61–65; through props, 12–47
Integration—post-savasana reflection, 51–53
Iyengar, B.K.S.—on savasana difficulty, xiv, 10, 83, 88

Jaw and tongue—softening cues, 15
Joy—natural outcome of letting go, 93

Karma—continuity of self and rebirth, 82, 84–86
Keller, Doug—on rolling to the right, 55

Lasater, Judith—rolling to either side, 55–56
Laya yoga—dissolution practice, 4
Left-side savasana—for pregnancy and digestion, 42–44
Letting go—paradox of non-doing, 48; surrender into death, 91–93
Light—as awareness or "blue pearl," 50
Little, Tias—threshold teachings, ix–xi, 57–58

Makarasana (sea-monster pose)— prone variation, 39–42
Mantra—repetition and inner sound, 66–68
Mind—quieting of, 8, 9–10, 48, 51; witness to thought, 51
Mudras— accessibility adaptations, 77; hand gestures and energies, 69–77
Muktananda, Swami—blue pearl teaching, 50

Nadis— cooling lunar current activated when rolling right, 55; energy channels, 69
Non-doing—essence of savasana, 48
Nose awareness—breath through nostrils, 55

Om—primordial vibration, 67–68
Open awareness—witnessing without control, 48

Paffard, Mary—on rolling left, 56
Patel, Ramanand—teaching stories and humor, 17, 20, 50, 52, 83, 90
Peace—arising from stillness, xi, 82
Pelvic floor—connection to breath, 16, 72, 73–74
Prana—life-force energy, 69–70
Pratyahara—in prone savasana, 39–42; withdrawal of senses, 62
Props—blankets, bolsters, sandbags, chairs, 10–11, 12–13, *various savasanas*

Raoult, François—on resonance and stillness, 9, 96, 107
Rebirth—cyclical view of self, 83–84
Reclining bound angle pose (supta baddha konasana)—restorative variation, 36–39
Rest—active and dynamic stillness, 10, 51–53
Rolling to the right—energetics and interpretations, 55, 56–57

Sacrum—alignment and support, 13
Sandbags—therapeutic uses on thighs, shoulders, forehead, 10, *various savasanas*
Sanskrit—pronunciation and transliteration, 6
Savasana—as daily meditation, ix, 4; historical roots, 3; mental state of, 51–53; physical setup, *various savasanas*; as practice of dying, 91–93
    classic supine form—foundational pose, 12–20
    eye wrap—to soothe and contain energy, 47
    prone savasana (makarasana)—psoas release and sensory withdrawal, 39–42
    reclining bound angle pose (supta baddha konasana)—restorative heart opener, 36–39
    seated savasana in a chair—for limited mobility, 45–47
    side-lying savasana (parsva savasana)—for pregnancy or back pain, 42–44
    supported with chair—for low back relief, 32–35
    with weight on forehead—to calm mind, 28–32
    with weight on humeri—for shoulder release, 25–27
    with weight on thighs—to release psoas, 21–24
Self— liberation of, 86; witnessing and dissolution of ego, xiv, 67–68
Spiritual—merging with, 67–78, 84, 86, 89, 104
Stillness—cultivating, 51–53; doorway to awareness, 89; dynamic, x
Surrender— letting go into grace, 91–93; nature of, 51–53

Teachers—guidance and lineage, 88, 126
Tongue and jaw—relaxation cues, 15
Transition—life-death continuum, 82, 87–89
Trust—inner knowing, 56

Unconscious—accessed through breath, 17, 66–68
Upanishads—philosophical background, 68, 108
Uplift—energetic rebound after rest, 72

Vayus—five vital winds, 62, 69
Vishuddha (throat chakra)—expression and surrender, 71, 76–77
Visualization—early 20th-century methods of savasana, 10–11

Weight variations—on forehead, 28–32; on humeri, 25–26; on thighs, 21–24
Witness consciousness—observing without judgment, 81–90

Yoga—as embodied philosophy, xiv, 3–4; meaning and evolution, 3–8
Yoga of Death—savasana as preparation for dying, 82, 87–89
Yogendra, Shri—early 20th-century teacher, 4–8

ABOUT THE AUTHORS

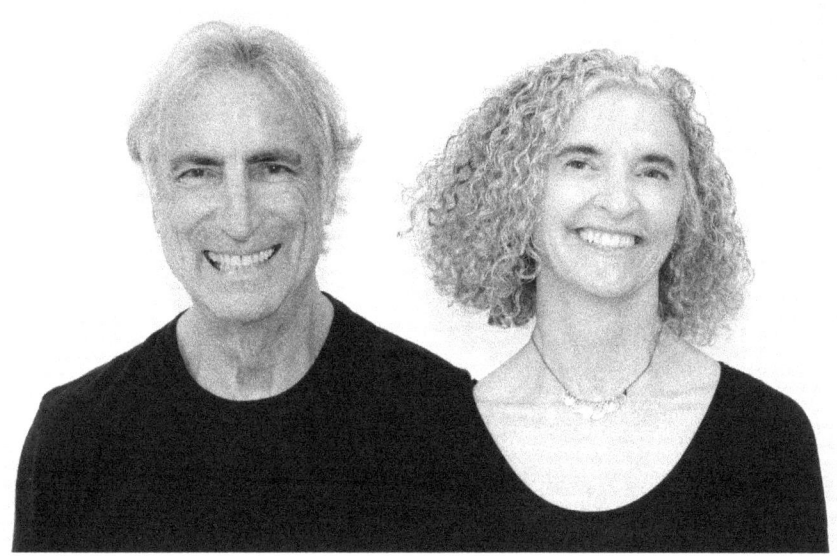

Leslie Howard is an Oakland-based yoga educator, author, and international workshop leader, best known for her pioneering work on pelvic floor health. She is the author of *Pelvic Liberation* and has taught thousands of students and teachers worldwide how to connect with the wisdom and complexity of the female pelvis.

Her deep dive into savasana began with profound experiences in this underappreciated pose and gradually expanded into broader questions about embodiment, stillness, and mortality.

Leslie is a trained hospice volunteer with Kaiser Permanente and a certified death doula, bringing years of end-of-life care experience into her teaching and writing. Her work bridges yoga, anatomy, contemplative care, and subtle-body philosophy, offering a compassionate and grounded approach to both living and dying. She has designed two successful studies with the University of California, San Francisco on yoga for incontinence and pelvic pain, and is a longtime contributor and presenter for *Yoga Journal*.

To learn more about Leslie, visit: www.lesliehowardyoga.com

Richard Rosen began his yoga practice in 1980 and completed his two-year teacher training in 1984 at the BKS Iyengar Yoga Institute in San Francisco. In 1987, with his good friend Rodney Yee, he co-founded the Piedmont Yoga Studio in Oakland. Richard has served on the boards of *Yoga Journal* magazine, for which he was also a contributing editor, and its offshoot, Yoga Dana, an organization that provided grants to teachers working with physically disabled students and students in prisons, juvenile centers, halfway houses, and more. Richard has published six books on yoga, the most recent being *Yoga by the Numbers: The Sacred & Symbolic in Yoga Philosophy and Practice* (2022). He has also contributed articles and reviews to a number of yoga magazines, especially *Yoga Journal*. Richard lives in beautiful Berkeley, California, in a cottage built in 1906.

www.ingramcontent.com/pod-product-compliance
Lightning Source LLC
Chambersburg PA
CBHW040004040426
42337CB00033B/5217